THE HEALTHCARE SUPERVISOR

EFFECTIVE COMMUNICATION

Edited by
Charles R. McConnell
Vice President for Employee Affairs
The Genesee Hospital
Rochester, New York

AN ASPEN PUBLICATION®
Aspen Publishers, Inc.
Gaithersburg, Maryland
1993

Library of Congress Cataloging-in-Publication Data

The health care supervisor on effective communication/ [edited by]
Charles R. McConnell.
p. cm.
Articles originally published in the health care supervisor.
Includes bibliographical references and index.
ISBN: 0-8342-0365-0
1. Health facilities — Personnel management.
2. Communication in personnel management.
3. Supervision of employees. I. McConnell,
Charles R. II. Health care supervisor.
[DNLM: 1. Health Facility Administrators—collected works.
2. Communication—collected works.
3. Personnel Management—methods—collected works.
WX 159 H434 1993]
RA971.35.H423   1993
362. 1'1' 0683—dc20
DNLM/DLC
for Library of Congress
93-198
CIP

Aspen Publishers, Inc. grants permission for photocopying for limited personal or internal use. This consent does not
extend to other kinds of copying, such as copying for general distribution, for advertising or promotional purposes, for
creating new collective works, or for resale. For information, address
Aspen Publishers, Inc., Permissions Department, 200 Orchard Ridge Drive, Suite 200,
Gaithersburg, Maryland 20878.

Editorial Resources: Barbara Priest

Library of Congress Catalog Card Number: 93-198
ISBN: 0-8342-0365-0

Printed in Canada

1 2 3 4 5

Contents

Part I   The Communication Environment

Part II Ups and Downs in Organizational Communication

Part III   Self-Help for the Supervisor

Part IV   Of Problems and Groups

Preface

INTRODUCTION

The Health Care Supervisor is a cross-disciplinary journal that publishes articles of relevance to persons who manage the work of others in health care settings. This journal's readers, as well as its authors, come from a wide variety of functional, clinical, technical, and professional backgrounds. Between the covers of a single issue of *HCS*, for example, you can find articles written by a nurse, a physician, a speech pathologist, a human resource specialist, an accountant, a nursing home administrator, and an attorney. These authors, and the numerous others who write for *HCS*, write with a single purpose: to provide guidance that all health care supervisors, regardless of the occupations or specialties they supervise, can use in learning to better understand or fulfill the supervisory role.

Very nearly all of the articles appearing in *HCS* could be described as dealing in some way with effective communication. In a very real sense, the essence of supervising *is* communication. The supervisor is charged with ensuring that certain work gets done, more work than one person could accomplish alone. To get this work done the supervisor must fully communicate to a number of employees how it is to be done, when it must be done, and numerous details concerning the organization and its functioning. Similarly, the supervisor must function as a link in the interdepartmental communication processes that keep the entire organization going in its chosen direction. Because supervising is about getting things accomplished through other people, supervising is also about communicating with those people.

Every issue or two, however, perhaps two or three times each year, *HCS* runs an article devoted specifically to the problems and processes of communication in the setting of the workplace. In, *The Health Care Supervisor on Effective Communication*, we have collected 21 articles that address dimensions of communication within the workplace as it may concern the supervisor. Encompassed by these articles are matters of organizational culture and environment; barriers to communication; listening and nonverbal processes; meetings, committees, and other group processes; and the all-important supervisor–employee relationship.

THE COMMUNICATION ENVIRONMENT

In "Organizational Climate in the Health Care Setting," Munn reminds us that the environment in which one communicates can greatly influence what flows among persons. Pozgar aptly points out in "Perceptive Communications" that effective communication runs far deeper than mere words or audible messages, and with "Sexist Language in Health Care Facilities" DiGaetani interjects some essential advice concerning the necessity of taking all sexist connotations out of the spoken and written language of business.

UPS AND DOWNS IN ORGANIZATIONAL COMMUNICATION

"The Supervisor's Central Role in Organizational Communication" appropriately places the first-line manager in the center of the action, with strong communications responsibilities upward, downward, and laterally. As if tridirectional communication responsibilities were not enough, in "On the Grapevine" Pozgar describes the workings of the countless other channels that flow around us and, in only some instances, include us.

In "Health Care Supervisors Identify Communication Barriers in Their Supervisor–Subordinate Relationships," Golen and Boissoneau present some study result that can help supervisors recognize the obstacles most commonly encountered between employee and supervisor.

The three-part series, "Making Upward Communication Work For Your Employees," examines a variety of ways of getting information to move in the direction that produces the most natural resistance to communication. These include means as informal as the simple "open door" and as extensive and formal as employee attitude surveys.

In "Overcoming Barriers to True Two-Way Communication With Employees" the supervisor is guided in recognizing and avoiding the principal obstacles to the establishment of sound supervisor-employee relationships.

SELF HELP FOR THE SUPERVISOR

The overriding theme of this part is *how to*, beginning with how to relate on a basic, friendly, person-to-person level as in Brown's "Improving Communication: The Use of Management Parables" and how to sharpen one's listening skills, as described by Munn in "The Supervisor as a Responsible Listener."

Munn continues with "Not By Words Alone," telling us how to recognize nonverbal cues and otherwise tune in to wordless messages.

In "Interviewing Skills: Selecting the Right Candidate," Metzger guides us through the all-important process of selecting employees. In another critical application of the one-on-one contact, Mancision explores the employee evaluation discussion in "The Appraisal Interview: Constructive Dialogue in Action."

"A Giant Step Toward Improved Supervisory Effectiveness" suggests how to solidify working relationships with employees and increase one's own effectiveness with the use of simple deadlines and follow up.

OF PROBLEMS AND GROUPS

We are reminded by Bertinasco in "Strategies for Resolving Conflict" that disagreements and differences within groups of people are inevitable and must be addressed. Snook and Umiker examine conflict and more in "Advantages and Disadvantages of Committees" and "How to Generate Power in Meetings," respectively, guiding the supervisor in working with these frequently essential but sometimes runaway processes that possess the potential for generating the best and the worst of group communication.

In "Running Small Meetings: An Overlooked Technique for Making Them Productive and Keeping Them Short," Nelson and Saunders suggest the limited use of formal meeting procedures for the sake of brevity and productivity. Finally, in "Creating Opportunities for Employee Participation in Problem Solving' Kahn overviews some of the techniques available for bringing employees together on common interests and concerns.

CONCLUSION

The Health Care Supervisor on Effective Communication contains a great deal of information that can help the supervisor become a better communicator and thus a better manager. First and foremost in improving one's facility at communication, however, is the desire to improve as a communicator, to minimize problems owing to misunderstanding or lack of information, and to generally do a better job of managing people. For the sincerely interested individual, the authors represented in this book offer tried and proven practical advice.

Acknowledgments

It would not have been possible to assemble this volume without the active involvement of the members of the guiding boards, past and present of The Health Care Supervisor. As of this writing some of these valued advisors and authors are well into their second decade of service to HCS. Our sincere thanks to the past members of the HCS Editorial Board, the present HCS Advisory Board, and the present Board of Contributing Editors.

Past Members of Editorial Board

Steven H. Appelbaum, Zeila W. Bailey, Claire D. Benjamin, Marjorie Beyers, Philip Bornstein, Leonard C. Brideau, Robert W. Broyles, Joy D. Calkin, Kenneth P. Cohen, Joseph A. Cornell, Darlene A Dougherty, Kenneth R. Emery, Valerie Glesnes-Anderson, Lee Hand, Allen G. Herkimer, Jr., Max G. Holland, Bowen Hosford, Charles E. Housley, Laura L. Kalick, Janice M. Kurth, Loucine M. D. Huckabay, Marlene Lamnin, Joan Gratto Liebler, Ellyn Luros, Margeurite, R. Mancini, Robert D. Miller, Joan F. Moore, Victor J. Morano, Harry E. Munn, Jr., Michael W. Noel, Rita E. Numerof, Samuel E. Oberman, Cheryl S. O'Hara, Jesus J. Pena, Donald J. Petersen, Tim Porter-O'Grady, George D. Pozgar, Ann Marie Rhodes, Edward P Richards III, James C. Rose, Rachel Rotkovich, Norton M. Rubenstein, Edward D. Sanderson, William L. Scheyer, Homer H., Schmitz, Joyce L. Schweiger, Donna Richards Sheridan, Margaret D. Sovie, Eugene I. Stearns, Judy Ford Stokes, Thomas J. Tenerovicz, Lewis H. Titterton, Jr., Dennis A Tribble, Terry Trudeau, Alex J. Vallas, Katherine W. Vestal, Judith Weilerstein, William B. Werther, Jr., Shirley Ann Wertz, Sara J. White, Norman H. Witt, and Karen Zander

Present HCS Advisory Board

Addison C. Bennett, Bernard L. Brown, Jr., Karen H. Henry, Norman Metzger, I. Donald Snook, Jr., and Helen Yura-Petro

Board of Contributing Editors

Donald F. Back, Robert Boissoneau, Jerad D. Browdy, Vicki S. Crane, Carol A Distasio, Charlotte Eliopoulos, Howard L. Lewis, R. Scott MacStravic, Leon McKenzie, Jerry L. Norville, Stephen L. Priest, Howard L. Smith, and John L. Templin, Jr.

Our sincere appreciation as well to those who, in addition to the persons mentioned above, participated in creating the articles that make up this volume:

Linda Bertinasco, John L. DiGaetani, Steven Golen, Susan Kahn, Jeanne Mancision, Marianna Nelson, Zane Saunders, and William Umiker.

Part I
The Communication Environment

Organizational climate in the health care setting

Harry E. Munn, Jr.
Associate Professor
Department of Speech
   Communication
North Carolina State University
Raleigh, North Carolina

WHAT IS organizational climate? This question can best be answered with an analogy. Organizational climate is both similar to and different from the weather. The weather affects not only our physical comfort, but also our behavior and therefore our relationships with other people.

R. Wayne Pace tells us that the communication climate of an organization affects the way we work: to whom we talk, whom we like, how we feel, how hard we work, how innovative we are, what we want to accomplish and how we seem to fit into the organization.[1]

For further clarification of organizational climate, consider the following metaphorical description provided by Halpin. In this description one could easily substitute hospital, clinic, nursing home or any other type of health care facility for the word *school.*

Health Care Superv, 1984,3(1),19–29
© 1984 Aspen Publishers, Inc.

Anyone who visits more than a few schools notes quickly how schools differ from each other in their *feel*. In one school the teachers and students are zestful and exude confidence in what they are doing. They find pleasure in working with each other; this pleasure is transmitted to the students, who thus are given at least a fighting chance to discover that school can be a happy experience. In a second school the brooding discontent of the teachers is palpable; the principal tries to hide his incompetence and his lack of sense of direction behind a cloak of authority, and yet he wears his cloak poorly because the attitudes he displays toward others vacillate randomly between the obsequious and the officious. And the psychological sickness of such a faculty spills over on the students who, in their own frustration, feed back to the teachers a mood of despair. A third school is neither marked by joy nor despair, but by hollow ritual. Here one gets the feeling of watching an elaborate charade in which teachers, principal, and students are acting out parts. The acting is smooth, even glib, but it appears to have little meaning for the participants; in a strange way the show doesn't seem to be for real. And so, too, as one moves to other schools, one finds that each appears to have a *personality* of its own. It is this personality that we describe here as organizational climate of the school.[2]

Similarly, the organizational climate of a hospital is not something that one can directly see or touch. We can nevertheless sense it just as easily as a nurse or physician can sense that something is wrong with a patient. Though no thermometer can measure it, the organizational climate can be changed. People create their own work environment; if it is not right, people can change it, and the health care supervisor can be an important agent of change as he or she attempts to help alter the climate in a positive direction.

Evans defines organizational climate as "a multidimensional perception by members, as well as nonmembers, of the essential attributes or character of an organizational system."[3] He goes on to make the following assumptions about organizational climate.

- Members as well as nonmembers have perceptions about the climate of the organization.
- Organizational members tend to perceive the climate differently than nonmembers because of their prevalence of different frames of reference and different criteria for evaluating the organization.
- Perceptions of organizational climate, whether real or unreal, have behavioral consequences for the organization as well as for the organization-set, i.e., the complement of organizations with which the organization interacts.
- Organizational members performing differing roles tend to have different perceptions of the climate, if only because of (1) a lack of role census, (2) a lack of uniformity in role socialization and (3) a diversity in patterns of role-set interactions.
- Members of different organizational subunits tend to have dif-

ferent perceptions of the climate because of different role-set configurations, different subgoals and different subcommitments to the goals of subunits compared to the goals of the organization as a whole.[4]

Thus, the eye of the beholder plays a key role in determining organizational climate. How health care employees see their roles and the roles of others in the organization helps to determine whether the climate is positive or negative.

GROUP CLIMATE

The importance of a positive group climate should not be underestimated by the health care supervisor. Redding states, "The climate of an organization is more critical than the communication skills or techniques (taken by themselves) in creating an effective organization."[5]

Sociological dimensions of climate

There are six sociological dimensions of climate. By applying these to their jobs, supervisors can increase their effectiveness as motivational agents of change.

Clarity

Clarity refers to the supervisor's sense of understanding of the hospital's goals and policies. This requires an effort to make things run smoothly, as opposed to an acceptance of confusion. Supervisors will change the or-

ganizational climate in a positive direction if they

- see that information flows smoothly;
- help their employees plan and organize activities; and
- help their employees to understand what is expected of them.

Patton and Giffin believe that the importance of goal specificity cannot be overemphasized. Their work has led them to believe that groups fail, lose member commitment, bog down and develop interpersonal dislikes because of a lack of specific goal identification.[6] Their point is that if you aim for nothing in particular, it is likely that you will achieve just that.

Commitment

Supervisors must have a continuing commitment to goal achievement. This commitment is related to acceptance of realistic goals, an involvement in goal setting and a continuous evaluation of performance compared to goals. Supervisors will change the organizational climate in a positive direction if

- they involve their employees in goal setting and review meetings;
- their employees recognize the goals and consider them to be realistic and meaningful; and
- their employees have a personal commitment to achieve the goals.

Goodson describes a group as a small social system. It consists of persons influencing and being influenced by one another and attracted to the same or similar concerns, goals and values. Group goals can only be achieved when there is a relatively high degree of group consensus.[7]

Standards

Here the focus is on the emphasis that the supervisor places on setting high standards of performance. Supervisors will change the organizational climate in a positive direction if they

- set tough and challenging personal goals;
- can instill pride in doing a job well; and
- are interested in improving individual performance.

Zander has found that a group's aspiration level helps to determine its degree of success or failure.

After repeated success, members who perceive that the future promises a greater likelihood of success at that level of difficulty, raise their anticipated level of aspiration, develop feelings of success and pride in the group, assign a favorable evaluation to their group's performance, attribute greater value to future success, develop a disposition to seek further success, perceive their group to be an attractive one, and become committed to the process of setting future goals. Individuals who have more responsible positions are more likely to have the reactions just described than are those with less important roles.

On the other hand, after repeated failure, members are less inclined to be concerned about the probabilities of future failure, or success; instead, they seek means that will help them avoid the unfa-

vorable consequences of failure. They tend to: lower the group's goal or stick to the one they have failed to reach, give an unapproving evaluation of their group's performance, see the activity as less important, believe that success in the task is less desirable, are less attracted to their own group and would like to judge the group in relation to its past performance rather than goal attainment. They would gladly abandon altogether the practice of setting aspiration levels. Members of such groups have a distinct preference for unreasonably difficult tasks, in light of their past performance, making them highly vulnerable to subsequent failure.[8]

Responsibility

This dimension concerns the supervisor's feelings of personal responsibility for work, involving a sense of autonomy stemming from both real delegation and encouragement to take individual initiatives. Supervisors will change the organizational climate in a positive direction if they:

- feel they can help employees solve problems;
- encourage themselves and their employees to take increased responsibility; and
- help employees to develop a sense of independence and to feel the employees' judgment is trusted.

Haney questioned 6,000 supervisors in 43 organizations of various types and sizes. The overwhelming majority believed that high trust tended to stimulate high performance. The supervisors felt that subor-

---

When the organizational climate can be characterized as trusting and supportive, communication will be improved.

---

dinates generally responded well to their confidence in them. When the organizational climate can be characterized as trusting and supportive, communication will also be improved.[9]

Recognition

Supervisors must feel that they and their employees will be recognized for doing a good job. They should not feel that criticism is more likely than recognition for good performance. Supervisors will change the organizational climate in a positive direction if

- their employees see rewards related to excellence of performance;
- their employees see the existence of a promotion system that helps the best person to rise to the top; and
- they help their employees to see that rewards and recognition outweigh threats and criticism.

Harnack and Fest did a study that examined the small group behavior between effective and ineffective groups, making the following comparisons.

Effective groups have a high degree of permissiveness. This climate of permissiveness gives members an opportunity

to speak their minds; they are inhibited only by normal restrains of tact, propriety, and common sense. Members of ineffective groups exhibit the opposite behavior and act restrained during meetings. They leave the meeting muttering to themselves about the ideas they did not feel free to express. The effective group assigns tasks on the basis of people's skills and interests. The ineffective group assigns tasks with little thought or planning. Effective groups exhibit intergroup status where all members share in the recognition and rewards of group achievement. To become effective groups need successes and from successes the group builds confidence and is able to meet new challenges.[10]

Teamwork

Hospital supervisors and employees must feel that they belong to a health care team. This feeling is characterized by cohesion, mutual warmth, support, trust and pride. Supervisors will change the organizational climate in a positive direction if

- they help their employees to achieve mutual understanding and support;
- their employees see people trusting and respecting others; and
- they help their employees to develop a feeling of personal loyalty and a sense of belonging to their work group.

Jensen points to the fact that interdependency has a direct effect on a group member's sense of freedom to participate in the group process. If the member does not perceive or feel valued and accepted by others in the group, the member's emotional responses may lead to the restriction of his or her participation in the affairs of the group. A group member needs to feel approved, valued or esteemed by other group members. When this behavior is denied, the group member will drastically alter his or her behavior in order to avoid further loss.[11]

Environmental dimensions of climate

These environmental dimensions of climate combined with the sociological dimensions discussed earlier help to create a specific kind of organizational climate. The climate in which all employees discuss work problems is extremely important. The attractiveness of the meeting room, the intensity of lighting, table shape and seating arrangements all help to determine the type of work and communication that takes place within the small group.

Mehrabian notes the following:

The people who must be involved in organizational communication are the executives. The more important an executive is, the more critical it is that he or she be in the communication network. Yet, organizational arrangements work to produce the opposite effect. Important executives are inaccessible, while clerk typists are a part of virtually everything. It is small wonder, then, that studies of organizations repeatedly have found executives to know far less about organizational matters than do low level secretaries and clerks.[12]

This evidence suggests that few executives really know the true organizational climates of their work groups. As their isolation increases, their sensitivity to the sociological and environmental dimensions of climate decreases.

Room attractiveness

Maslow and Mintz (see Mintz[13]) studied three different types of rooms: one was an ugly room (designed to give the impression of a janitor's storeroom in a disheveled condition); one was an average room (a professor's office); and one was a beautiful room (complete with carpeting, drapes and other room accessories). They attempted to keep all factors such as time of day, type of seating, odor, noise and the experimenter constant from room to room so the results could be solely attributed to the type of room.

The ugly room was described as producing fatigue, monotony, discontent, sleep, irritability and hostility. On the other hand, the beautiful room produced feelings of pleasure, enjoyment, comfort, energy, importance and a desire to continue the activity.

Some hospitals and health care facilities are finding that aesthetics are extremely important to their patients' well-being. They are moving away from tiled floors and installing carpeting as a medium for humanizing the institutional environment. Greco reports that patients surveyed both in personal interviews and in a survey sent to their homes reacted favorably to the carpet found in the hospital.

Patients responded that the carpeting provided a more homelike atmosphere, that it was colorful, provided a feeling of warmth, seemed less noisy and made the hospital seem more spacious.[14]

Other studies by Cheek, Maxwell and Wiesman provided similar results. These researchers studied two psychiatric wards and in both cases found that the patients responded favorably to the presence of carpeting. The patients felt the carpeting was more comfortable, warmer, more homelike and made their ward seem less like a hospital.[15]

Illumination

More research needs to be conducted with respect to the levels of lighting related to group productivity and job satisfaction. The few studies that have been conducted seem to suggest that too much light or too little light does produce fatigue and that women seem to be less sensitive to glare than men are. The secret seems to be to find the right amount of light that is necessary to satisfactorily do the job. A mechanical task, for example, may require more light than is necessary for good interpersonal communication.

Kowinski surmises that, "Most offices are generally overlit, they have twice as much light as they need, while individuals within the office are working in conditions that are underlit. The results can be inefficiency, fatigue, and perhaps a sense of dislocation caused mostly by the St. Vitus dance that the pupil of the eye must do to cope."[16]

The round table

During the Vietnam War, the dispute over the size and shape of the negotiating table in Paris provided a classic example of the importance placed on environmental dimensions as they symbolize status or equality in establishing a specific type of climate necessary for the negotiations.

McCroskey, Larson and Knapp describe this incident:

The United States (US) and South Viet Nam (SVN) wanted a seating arrangement in which only two sides were identified. They did not want to recognize the National Liberation Front (NLF) as an *equal* party in the negotiations. North Viet Nam (NVN) and the NLF wanted *equal* status given to all parties—represented by a four sided table. The final arrangement was such that both parties could claim victory. The *round table* minus the dividing lines allowed North Viet Nam and the NLF to claim all four delegations were equal. The existence of the two secretarial tables (interpreted as dividers), the lack of identifying symbols on the table, and an AA, BB speaking rotation permitted the United States and South Viet Nam to claim victory for the two sided approach. Considering the amount of lives lost during the eight months needed to arrive at the seating arrangement, we can certainly conclude that territorial space has extremely high priority in some interpersonal settings.[17]

The round table, of course, goes back to the days of the Knights of the Round Table and is a graphic illustration of power. The table was round so that all of the knights could be seen as being equal. However, King Arthur's seat became the status marker and status decreased as the distance from the king increased. Thus the knights who sat close to the king were seen as having the higher status.

Koneya and Barbour state that the order of power at a round table is usually clockwise, beginning with the number 12 on a clock face. Power decreases as it moves around the table at 3 o'clock, 6 o'clock and 9 o'clock. Therefore, the second most powerful person will sit in the 1 o'clock position, and the least powerful will sit at the 11 o'clock position.[18]

The square table

Malandro and Barker suggest that the square table, with four equal sides, provides excellent corners for the separation of its participants. For a business meeting, the square table signifies equality for each business partner, since each individual has equal footage, space and separate edges. The square table also has an equal length on each side. However, because of distinct sidedness, it does not constitute unity. It is excellent for competition because it encourages direct eye contact in all four positions and allows for equal distance between the members seated at the table.[19]

The rectangular table

The most common and, for some reason, the most popular table used

for organizational meetings is the rectangular table. The most obvious reason for its popularity is that a large number of people can be gathered about the table. This also gives the group leader the opportunity to sit at the head of the table and be seen easily by his or her fellow employees.

Howells and Becker reasoned that spatial positions at the rectangular table would determine the flow of communication and consequently determine the degree of the individuals' status in the group. Some five-person decision-making groups, in which three people sat on one side of a rectangular table and two sat on the other side, were examined. The side with two people proved to be more influential because more communication was directed at them and this, consequently, enabled them to talk more. Communication at a rectangular table flows across the table rather than around it.[20]

Further studies conducted by Hare and Bales revealed that persons sitting at the ends or in the middle of a rectangular table have a higher talking frequency than members sitting in other positions.[21]

There is evidence to suggest that the seat in which one chooses to sit is no accident. Cook found that extroverts chose opposite seats or chose positions that would place them in close proximity of one another. Introverts, on the other hand, chose seats that would provide them with more distance from the dominant group members.[22] When attempting to establish a positive overall group cli-

Supervisory Climate Survey

Instructions

For each of the statements below draw a circle around one of the following: A—Always, F—Frequently, O—Occasionally, S—Seldom, N—Never.

For example, if you feel that you are frequently encouraged to come up with new and original ideas, you would circle the "F" in the following question:

A F O S N   1. We are encouraged to come up with new and original ideas.

Use only one evaluative letter code for each answer.

A F O S N   1. I have the opportunity to review my overall performance and effectiveness with my supervisor.

A F O S N   2. There is much respect between management and other personnel in this group.

A F O S N   3. In this organization, the rewards and encouragements you receive for effective performance outweigh the threats and criticisms.

A F O S N   4. Our people are encouraged to make decisions when the situation demands an immediate decision.

A F O S N   5. In this group, I am given a chance to participate in setting the performance goals for my job.

A F O S N   6. The rooms in which we hold meetings for decision making are conducive to good interpersonal communication.

A F O S N   7. I feel that I am a member of a well-functioning team.

A F O S N   8. My supervisor is easily accessible to all of his or her employees.

A F O S N   9. We are encouraged to come up with new and original ideas.

A F O S N   10. In this group we are rewarded in proportion to how well we do.

A F O S N   11. As a group we can disagree without becoming disagreeable.

A F O S N   12. People are proud to belong to this group.

A F O S N   13. In this group, what constitutes good performance has been identified.

A F O S N   14. Most of our meetings are held in attractive rooms.

A F O S N   15. The results I am supposed to achieve in my job are realistic.

A F O S N   16. In meetings we may sit wherever we wish.

A F O S N   17. In this group, people demonstrate strong commitment to achieving group performance.

A F O S N   18. Things seem to be well organized in my group.

A F O S N   19. There is good communicative balance in my group.

A F O S N   20. People in this group help each other in solving job-related problems.

A F O S N   21. In this group, people come to meetings well prepared.

A F O S N   22. We can disagree with our boss and not fear any form of reprisal.

A F O S N   23. I am involved in setting my own performance goals and in understanding how they relate to the overall goals of my group.

A F O S N   24. My supervisor does a good job in recognizing good performance.

A F O S N   25. Our overall organizational climate is a positive one.

Score the Supervisory Climate Survey in the following manner: Always, 4 points; Frequently, 3 points; Occasionally, 2 points; Seldom, 1 point; Never, 0 points.

Your organizational climate is excellent if you scored 90 to 100 points, good if you scored 80 to 89 points, average if you scored 70 to 79 points, fair if you scored 60 to 69 points and poor if you scored less than 60 points.

mate, the health care supervisor has to find a method whereby the quieter members of the group can be encouraged to participate or the group will never realize its full potential.

The decision to spend time improving the organizational climate within health care work groups is one that supervisors must make for themselves. Remember, organizational climate does not just happen. Rather, it is the collective view of the people within an organization as to the nature of the environment in which they work, and they can make that climate anything they want it to be. Highly motivated individuals tend to work in supportive organizational climates. We live in climates of our own making, and these self-made climates affect our relationships with others.

The organizational climate extends into every unit of the health care facility. No one can see it or touch it, but every health care employee or patient can sense it. When employees sense a supportive organizational climate, it reaffirms their basic reason for being and for caring about people and improved patient care.

A SUPERVISORY CLIMATE SURVEY

The supervisory climate survey in the boxed insert is aimed at gaining a better understanding of the kind of work climate or environment in which your employees work, of the way in which the climate is created, and how it affects job performance and ultimately the job satisfaction of the employee.

As you fill out the questionnaire, respond to the items as they relate to your health care work group. *Do not* assume that pay, money or economic gains are implied by any of the questions. That is, questions that deal with recognition assume nonfinancial recognition.

Finally, if most health care supervisors and employees could only remember the following, they would be taking a giant step toward the development of a supportive organizational climate within their health care facility:

The Six Most Important Words
I ADMIT I MADE A MISTAKE
The Five Most Important Words
YOU DID A GOOD JOB
The Four Most Important Words
WHAT IS YOUR OPINION?
The Three Most Important Words
IF YOU PLEASE
The Two Most Important Words
THANK YOU
The One Most Important Word
WE
The Least Important Word
I

(anonymous)

REFERENCES

1. Pace, R. *Organizational Communication.* Englewood Cliffs, N.J.: Prentice-Hall, 1983, p. 125.

2. Halpin, A. *Theory and Research in Administration.* New York: Macmillan, 1966, p. 131.

3. Evans, W. *Organizational Theory: Structures,*

Systems, and Environment. New York: Wiley, 1976, p. 137.

4. Ibid., 139.

5. Redding, C. *Communication within the Organization: An Interpretive Review of Theory and Research.* New York: Industrial Communication Council, 1972, p. 111.

6. Patton, B. and Giffin, K. *Problem Solving Group Interaction.* New York: Harper & Row, 1973, p. 147–48.

7. Goodson, M. "The Person and the Group in American Culture and Education." In *The Dynamics of Instructional Groups*, edited by N. Henry. Chicago: University of Chicago Press, 1960, p. 15.

8. Zander, A. *Motives and Goals in Groups.* New York: Academic Press, 1971, p. 174.

9. Haney, W. *Communication and Interpersonal Relations: Text and Cases.* (Homewood, Ill.: Irwin, 1979, p. 13.

10. Harnack, V.R., and Fest, T.B. *Group Discussion Theory and Technique.* New York: Appleton-Century-Crofts, 1964, p. 181.

11. Jensen, G. "The Sociopsychological Structure of the Instructional Group." In *The Dynamics of Instructional Groups*, edited by N. Henry. Chicago: University of Chicago Press, 1960, p. 97.

12. Mehrabian, A. *Public Places and Private Spaces.* New York: Basic Books, 1976, p. 82.

13. Mintz, N.L. "Effects of Esthetic Surroundings: II. Prolonged and Repeated Experience in a 'Beautiful' and 'Ugly' Room." *Journal of Psychology* 41 (April 1956): 459–66.

14. Greco, J.T. "Carpeting vs. Resilient Flooring." *Hospitals* 39, no. 12 (1965): 55–58.

15. Cheek, F., Maxwell, R., and Wiesman, R. "Carpeting the Ward: An Exploratory Study in Environmental Psychiatry." *Mental Hygiene* 55 (January 1971): 109–18.

16. Kowinski, W. "Shedding New Light." *New Times* (March 7, 1975): 48.

17. McCroskey, J.C., Larson, C.E., and Knapp, M.L. *An Introduction to Interpersonal Communication.* Englewood Cliffs, NJ: Prentice-Hall, 1971, p. 98.

18. Koneya, M., and Barbour, A. *Louder than Words . . . Nonverbal Communication.* Columbus, Ohio: Charles E. Merrill, 1976, pp. 58–59.

19. Malandro, L.A., and Barker, L. *Nonverbal Communication.* Reading, Mass.: Addison-Wesley, 1983, p. 194.

20. Howells, L.T., and Becker, S.W. "Seating Arrangement and Leadership Emergence." *Journal of Abnormal and Social Psychology* 64 (February 1962): 148–50.

21. Hare, A., and Bales, R. "Seating Position and Small Group Interaction." *Sociometry* 26 (December 1963): 480–86.

22. Cook, M. "Experiments on Orientation and Proxemics." *Human Relations* 23 (February 1970): 61–76.

Perceptive communications

George D. Pozgar
Administrator
St. John's Episcopal Hospital
Smithtown, New York

For good or ill, your conversation is your advertisement. Every time you open your mouth, you let men look into your mind. Do they see it well-clothed, neat, businesslike?[1]

COMMUNICATION can be a pleasant and delightful experience. It can also be distasteful and annoying. Perceptive communication, the ability to convey or receive information with understanding, is the most written about and talked about but least understood management topic. It is a perennial subject presented at numerous lectures, conferences and seminars by a wide variety of professional groups.

The ability to express oneself orally and in writing is a skill that is required repeatedly of college-bound students, job applicants and those who aspire to climb the ladder of success. It is a skill desired by all and conquered by few. Those who have acquired this skill are generally suc-

Health Care Superv, 1983,1(4),1–13
© 1983 Aspen Publishers, Inc.

cessful in motivating others. The politician who is able to convince his or her constituency that his or her cause is just will remain in office. The supervisor who is able to communicate effectively with subordinates will be a successful motivator and will, in turn, enhance job satisfaction and goal attainment. Effective communication implies not only that the message is understood but also that the receiver is appropriately motivated to carry out instructions.

COMMUNICATION PROBLEMS

The problems of effective communication have existed since the creation of the first man and woman. Just as Eve trusted her first impression regarding the serpent's temptation that eating the fruit of a certain tree would make her and Adam "as gods, knowing good and evil" (Genesis 3:1–24), each person often accepts first impressions as reality. It takes time for individuals to understand one another, and it seems that few are willing to make that commitment.

Both supervisors and subordinates tend to perceive each new experience as reinforcing preconceived notions and biases and at the same time screening out those things that do not strengthen their ideas or individual conceptions of what the real world is all about. There is a tendency to make value judgments from one's own "frame of reference" and to evaluate all new knowledge according to its positive or negative impact on pre-established beliefs.

The key to success in management is the ability to listen, to understand and to respond appropriately to communications. The communication of thoughts and ideas is made possible by a common language. Although the spoken word is not the only method of conveying a thought or idea, it is the most useful and sophisticated method. Human beings are the only mammals that have developed the ability to communicate by spoken language. Can you imagine how difficult it would be if the supervisor or subordinate would have to act out a message, as do certain species of bees, which by means of a complex dance explain the location of nearby nectar?

Body language, such as posture and how one crosses arms or legs, may reveal a person's attitude but at the same time provide very little other useful information. However, this is not to imply that the supervisor should ignore the unspoken reactions that occur during the process of communication.

The process of communication is more difficult in multilingual and multicultural environments. A simple whistle may be a gesture of approval in one culture, whereas it is a sign of disapproval in another. The various dialects and semantic differences within a given language further complicate the process of meaningful communication.

Health services, and the number of specialized personnel and regulations affecting each new service, have grown at a tremendous rate during the past several decades. Hospital departments are developing an ever increasing interdependency for proper functioning (e.g., the intensive care unit depends on purchasing for supplies, central supply for sterile instruments, laboratory for test results, maintenance for proper lighting and heating, and personnel for employees). This interdependency creates a need for effective communication.

When communication is inadequate, complaints will subtly materialize in the various services. For example:

1. Bill did not get the message about the new sick leave policy. Jerry received the message but did not understand it. As a result, Jerry conveyed incorrect information to employees within his department. Carol got the information but failed to pass it along to the supervisors in her department. Nancy received the information but misplaced it.

2. Phil in maintenance notified May in nursing and John in x-ray that all electrical power would be shut off in the north wing of the hospital. The power was scheduled for shut-off from 8:00 A.M. to 10:00 A.M. on Saturday, November 10, 1982, so that a new emergency generator for the north wing could be installed. Phil failed to notify the laboratory and, as a result of complications, had to reschedule the installation.

3. Jim received new regulations from the state health department. He distributed copies to all department heads with the exception of housekeeping. The housekeeper was disturbed because she obtained a copy from another department and learned that certain regulations pertained to her department. She felt that her division was the last to learn about the new regulations and that she should have personally received a copy of the regulations from the administrator.

4. Jill, the director of social services, was not notified until December 2, 1982, about a survey by the Joint Commission on Accreditation of Hospitals to be conducted at the hospital on December 4, 1982. On November 5 she had scheduled a vacation to begin on December 3. Jill was disturbed that she had not been notified earlier regarding the survey. She found out from Pam, the coffee shop supervisor, that notification of the survey was sent to the hospital early in November.

The foregoing examples illustrate the costliness of inadequate communication in an organization. The benefits of competent communication can be rewarding from both a financial and employee morale point of view.

Poor communication between a supervisor and a subordinate is transmitted quickly via the grapevine. The employee who is unskillfully treated will likely become inefficient and cause disenchantment among peers. The damage that can result from unskillful communications is incalculable, and the supervisor may find that the poor communication experienced with one employee is compounded by its effect on other employees.

The supervisor may find that the poor communication experienced with one employee is compounded by its effect on other employees.

It is much more productive and much less frustrating to communicate effectively than it is to resolve the conflicts that can arise from failure to spend the time and effort to communicate competently. As noted by Patrick Delany, "Think all you speak, but speak not all you think. Thoughts are your own; your words are so no more."[2]

Language can raise many barriers to successful and meaningful communications. Many times, because of individual differences, idiosyncrasies and societal values, language can obscure the true intent of the communicator.

As a language evolves and technological advances emerge, various disciplines (e.g., business, law, medicine and data processing) begin to develop their own vocabularies, and thus the problems of effective communication are compounded. The effective supervisor must develop a sense of understanding of the various language models and be aware of the many problems that can arise in applying them in day-to-day communications.

The ability to effectively use a language as a means for transmitting ideas requires the supervisor to keep linguistically current and take new approaches to communicating with subordinates. The supervisor must be aware of the language limitations of subordinates. Otherwise, both may be tuned in on different linguistic wavelengths.

As one considers the many possible distortions that can take place in the process of communication, one begins to wonder how anyone ever understands others. The addition of multiple personalities in group conversations can give rise to an exponential growth in the distortion factor. One is led to believe that it must have been much easier to communicate during the Stone Age.

THE COMMUNICATIONS MODEL

Figure 1 is a model of the process of communication formation, transmission and translation. The reader should review the model carefully to obtain a general understanding of the complex nature of the communication process.

The development of one's character depends on many lifetime influences, such as language, education, religion, experiences (past, present and future), culture, environment, work and physical traits, as presented in the figure.

There are 16 selected individual personality and ability traits listed in the figure, which describe certain characteristics of a communicator (sender) and communicatee (receiver) at a stated time in their lives. The figure illustrates how each individual has developed each particular trait; for example, the communicator is an introvert and the communicatee is an extrovert. The percentiles at the top of the columns indicate the degree to which each person in the communication process has developed a specific trait.

It should be noted that ability and personality traits are not independent of one another. This is illustrated by the distortion grid in the figure. The distortion grid represents a melting pot for an individual's wants, needs and expectations. The interaction of the various traits within each individual acting on a given message at a given time can give rise to conflict, ideas, logic and so forth. It is of extreme importance for each party in a conversation to realize that one's response or reaction to another is significantly influenced by both lifetime influences and immediate life experiences, such as:

- What is my self-image?
- How do I feel (physical ailments)?
- Did I miss the train?
- Am I under pressure from my superiors to produce a report?
- Am I pressed for time?

- Did I have a good day or a bad day?
- Who am I communicating with—my superior, peer, subordinate, a stranger?

A message conceived of and conveyed by the communicator can be somewhat different from what is heard and understood by the communicatee and a third-party observer. The individual observing a two-way conversation generally recognizes more readily what message each party in the conversation is attempting to convey. That varying interpretations can be made of a message that has been transmitted illustrates the need for feedback, which in turn can be useful in developing a framework for understanding a message. Without such a framework, problem solving becomes more difficult because of intentional or unintentional distortions that can occur in the communication process.

Supervisors who do not provide a setting for feedback are providing the environment for an unmotivated and disgruntled staff. As one studies the model, it becomes quickly evident that there are literally thousands of factors that affect individuals' behavior and how they communicate.

Each party in a conversation should request clarification when he or she is not sure of the true intent of the message conveyed. Failure to request clarification can lead to misunderstandings and inappropriate actions. Just as there is a necessity to provide backup systems in national defense, computer operations and ac-

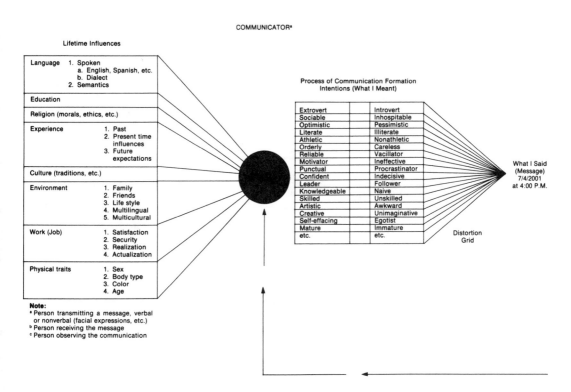

COMMUNICATOR[a]

Lifetime Influences

Language	1. Spoken
	a. English, Spanish, etc.
	b. Dialect
	2. Semantics

Education

Religion (morals, ethics, etc.)

Experience	1. Past
	2. Present time
	influences
	3. Future
	expectations

Culture (traditions, etc.)

Environment	1. Family
	2. Friends
	3. Life style
	4. Multilingual
	5. Multicultural

Work (Job)	1. Satisfaction
	2. Security
	3. Realization
	4. Actualization

Physical traits	1. Sex
	2. Body type
	3. Color
	4. Age

Note:
[a] Person transmitting a message, verbal
or nonverbal (facial expressions, etc.)
[b] Person receiving the message
[c] Person observing the communication

Process of Communication Formation
Intentions (What I Meant)

Extrovert	Introvert
Sociable	Inhospitable
Optimistic	Pessimistic
Literate	Illiterate
Athletic	Nonathletic
Orderly	Careless
Reliable	Vacillator
Motivator	Ineffective
Punctual	Procrastinator
Confident	Indecisive
Leader	Follower
Knowledgeable	Naive
Skilled	Unskilled
Artistic	Awkward
Creative	Unimaginative
Self-effacing	Egotist
Mature	Immature
etc.	etc.

Distortion
Grid

What I Said
(Message)
7/4/2001
at 4:00 P.M.

Figure 1. The process of communication.

count auditing, it is incumbent on each supervisor to be sure that he or she is acting on reliable information.

As a tool for communicating, language allows for the definition of observations that are necessary for organizing to achieve institutional goals and objectives. Language provides a means for individuals to understand one another and for describing a complex social system involving institutions, roles and expectations in general and each individual with his or her own personality, needs and dispositions in specific. The needs of both sides must be flexible.

The supervisor who can understand and apply these fundamental truths will be successful in developing the ability to turn crisis to advantage, deal with uncertainty, tolerate deviation, resolve conflict, encourage initiative and remain human under stress. Practical application of these sets of abilities is no easy task. If there were a perfect formula for dealing with such problems, there would

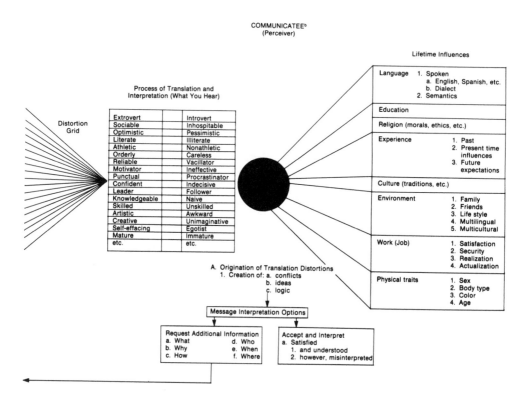

Figure 1. *(continued)*

be no need for innovative thinking on the process of communication.

Reality dictates that no two situations are exactly the same. The real world is in a constant state of flux, even though many times it is time and space that change at a more constant and reliable rate. Because the real world is undergoing continuing change, it is necessary to consistently strive to improve the communication process. The supervisor who has developed an understanding of the communication process and its short-

comings will not only be capable of operating within his or her own system of perception, but also be able to relate more effectively to his or her subordinates. The supervisor will then have the patience to develop a better understanding of himself or herself and others.

If an individual can accept the claim that no two individuals are the same, he or she will have come a long way in understanding the communication process. If the individual takes the time to understand, he or she will be much more effective and much less frustrated in interpersonal relationships both on the job and at home.

STEPS IN SUCCESSFUL COMMUNICATION

A key prerequisite for improving the communication process is for the supervisor to *want* to improve communication skills and overcome communication barriers. Changing poor communication habits is a full-time commitment. It cannot be an after-dinner or weekend pastime. Each and every communication setting must be considered a challenge to improve interpersonal relationships at home, work or play. As the supervisor begins to grasp the skills of meaningful conversation, he or she will find that good conversations bring self-fulfilling rewards.

Overcoming communication barriers

Conversation and dialogue must be a two-way street. The supervisor should encourage employee participation in the resolution of communication problems. The supervisor should also accept the idea that the real world may be different from how it is perceived and remember that individuals' perceptions of reality are programmed by past learnings.

The supervisor should provide a setting for open and informal as well as formal communications. He or she should generate an atmosphere of understanding. Each party in a conver-

sation should be put at ease. The supervisor should remember that the stress present in a given conversation causes a proportionate rise in the distortion factor. If a message is emotional, the supervisor should take time to clear the air. If a supervisor holds a meeting with an employee who appears to just want to ventilate, it may be better for the supervisor to reschedule the meeting.

If a message is not clear, the supervisor should request clarification. A message may have a completely different meaning when it is repeated. An employee's question should be rephrased to reassure the employee that his or her problem is understood

Perceptive communication

The supervisor should listen to an employee's communication and be tactful in response. The supervisor should not subconsciously prepare a response before the employee has completed the communication. The supervisor should realize that there is a constant need to understand others as well as himself or herself. Perceptive communication implies that one is able to observe and understand as well as be responsive. Caleb C. Colton, an English clergyman, is quoted as saying: "When in the company of sensible men, we ought to be doubly cautious of talking too much, lest we lose two things—their good opinions and our own improvement, for what we have to say we know, but what they have to say we know not."[3]

If the supervisor cannot give an appropriate response or an answer to a question, he or she should say so, but promise to get an answer. Improving perception and feedback will require some effort on the supervisor's part. Many inappropriate communication habits will have to be changed. The supervisor will never be perfect, but can strive for excellence.

Purposeful communication

Communications should have a purpose. The supervisor should ask himself or herself, what is it that I am trying to accomplish? The message the supervisor wishes to transmit must first be clear to him or her. Otherwise, the communication perceived by the employee will most likely be distorted. The supervisor should be precise and succinct and avoid transmitting irrelevant information. Such data will only hinder the communication process. Francois Rochefoucauld, a French moralist, is credited with saying: "As it is the characteristic of great wits to say much in few words, so it is of small wits to talk much, and say nothing."[4]

The supervisor should be precise and succinct and avoid transmitting irrelevant information.

It is just as important to avoid speaking incessantly as it is to listen intensely. Continuous talking tends to confuse the listener and lessen the listener's attention span, which in turn distorts the intended message.

The supervisor should communicate with a positive attitude. Negative feelings will only complicate the process, and little if anything will be accomplished.

The lines of communication must be open both horizontally (same level) and vertically (up and down) within the organization. There are many supervisors who believe they are communicating and seeking feedback when in reality they are expecting unquestioning obedience. Such supervisors purport to have an "open door policy" when in actuality the door is open only to those who reinforce their ideas. Supervisors with this management style will surround themselves with "yes men" (also known as toads, handshakers and apple polishers), who will in turn treat their subordinates in a like manner. Subordinates reporting to such superiors eventually become unmotivated and unproductive.

The supervisor should evaluate his or her own office. How is it perceived by subordinates? Is it a place of warmth and understanding, or is it cold and a place to be avoided? Whichever it is, the supervisor has created the atmosphere. Is it time to redecorate?

When hiring a new employee, the supervisor should explain the job and be open to questions. The supervisor should seek two-way communication. Communication failures often occur from the moment a prospective employee is hired. Each employee must clearly understand the mission of the organization and how his or her job contributes to achieving institutional goals and objectives. It is the role of the supervisor to effectively communicate this to the employee at the time of employment orientation and periodically throughout the year on a one-to-one basis. Regular departmental meetings should be conducted to provide an atmosphere for participation and understanding.

Supervisors with non-English-speaking employees will have to be innovative in the communication process (e.g., job descriptions and personnel handbooks can be written in Spanish). Employees who are bilingual can be helpful in the process of translation. Offering both English and non-English classes can also be beneficial in improving communications.

Effective communication

The supervisor should be selective in his or her choice of words when communicating. Words produce feelings. Words or phrases that tend to be inflammatory should be avoided. It should be remembered that a word or phrase that is acceptable to one person may be objectionable to another. The following quotations illustrate some notable and some regrettable comments from which all can learn.

President Ronald Reagan's choice of words on one occasion were "shut up." These words were considered appropriate for the occasion by some and inappropriate by others. The words *shut up* were probably the most publicized and, at the same time, the least important part of what he had to say. It is important to note that the communicatee in this instance clearly understood the message to "shut up" and sit down, which he did with haste and embarrassment. It is obviously much more difficult to speak extemporaneously under questioning by the press than when presenting a prepared speech or sermon.

Former President Jimmy Carter was asked at a television press conference to comment on his disagreement with Senator Edward Kennedy regarding the deregulation of oil prices. The president responded, "That's a lot of baloney." This comment did not make a good presentation for President Carter.

Former Secretary of State Alexander M. Haig, Jr. announced to reporters at a news conference following the attempted assassination of President Ronald Reagan that he was "in control here in the White House." This comment apparently annoyed Secretary of Defense Caspar W. Weinberger, who was of the opinion that he was in charge of operations in the White House Situation Room. The conflict as to who was in charge during the first hours following the assassination attempt created hard feelings among the rank and file party leaders. The moral of this story is "think before you speak."

President John F. Kennedy, during a dinner for Nobel prize winners, stated, "I think this is the most extraordinary collection of talent that has ever been gathered together at the White House with the possible exception of when Thomas Jefferson dined alone."

The following comments are quoted from President Kennedy's inaugural address: "I do not believe that any of us would exchange places with any other people or any other generation. The energy, the faith, the devotion which we bring to this endeavor will light our country and all who serve it. And the glow from that fire can truly light the world. And so, my fellow Americans, ask not what your country can do for you; ask what you can do for your country."

The Reverend Dr. Martin Luther King, Jr. in his address during his march in Washington, D.C. on August 28, 1963, stated, "I have a dream that one day this nation will rise up and live out the true meaning of its creed. We hold these truths to be self-evident that all men are created equal. I have a dream that one day on the red hills of Georgia the sons of former slaves and the sons of former slave owners will be able to sit down together at the table of brotherhood." The foregoing remarks by President John F. Kennedy and the Reverend Dr. Martin Luther King, Jr. illustrate the effectiveness of saying the right words at the right time.

Mayor Andrew Young, Ambassador to the United Nations when the United States was engaged in delicate negotiations with Britain about the future of Rhodesia, stated that the British had "practically invented rac-ism." Mayor Young is also noted as saying the Cubans "bring a certain stability to Angola," that there were "hundreds, maybe thousands of political prisoners" in the United States and that Ayatullah Khomeini would one day be viewed as "some kind of saint." These remarks lacked good communication etiquette, failed to follow appropriate rules of decorum and were not acceptable to society in general.

The foregoing quotations from press conferences, a social engagement and a sermon depict how one's communicative reactions can vary depending on the occasion. Some of the comments tended to invite anger and were obviously not an acceptable way to win friends and influence people. Others were compassionate and had a positive influence on the audience by creating an atmosphere of loyalty, fellowship and cooperation.

One's ability to communicate with dignity is certainly much easier when one is in the company of a sympathetic crowd than it is when one is in an antagonistic setting. The effective supervisor will not be a successful communicator on every occasion. However, the supervisor must not become discouraged and give up trying to improve communication skills just because of past inabilities to express himself or herself clearly.

There is most likely not a day that goes by in which one who engages in conversation cannot say "I spoke too much, I didn't say it right" or "I should have said more." When engaged in conversation, the supervisor should not hesitate to change course if it appears that it is going nowhere.

When engaged in conversation, the supervisor should not hesitate to change course if it appears that it is going nowhere.

Seldom does anyone participate in a conversation in which he or she is not aware of its effect on another. Failure to change course or direction midstream is many times a manifestation of stubbornness. As noted by John Casper Laveter, a Swiss theologian, "He who sedulously (persistently) attends, pointedly asks, calmly speaks, coolly answers and ceases when he has no more to say is in possession of some of the best requisites of conversation."[5]

The communication that takes place in group settings is often distorted by semantics. The supervisor must not assume that words mean the same things to different people. Not only do words mean different things to different people, but they also can have several definitions at different times. A 1940s statement that "John Doe is a flatfoot" implied that Mr. Doe had flat feet. A *flatfoot* in the 1960s was a slang word for police officer. The word *pot* (cooking utensil) is also a slang word for marijuana.

It is sufficiently difficult to cope with distortion caused by semantic differences during a one-to-one conversation. Add to that the semantical difficulties encountered during a group conversation with mixed ages, and one could end up constantly defining and redefining the intended message.

The effective supervisor must be aware that added meanings to words occur frequently at work. For example, the word *budget* could be defined by each department head in a given institution, and there would be a high probability that no two definitions would be exactly the same. The word *budget*, in the 1981 edition of Webster's *New Collegiate Dictionary*, is defined as:

a.) a statement of the financial position of an administration for a definite period of time based on estimates of expenditures during the period and proposals for financing them. b.) a plan for the coordination of resources and expenditures. c.) the amount of money that is available for, required for, or assigned to a particular purpose.

The word *budget*, in addition to its official definitions, can have many connotations and added meanings to different department heads, such as a great deal of hard work; the dollars actually available for the department during the budget year; the approved budget as a guideline within which the department must function; and an exercise in futility.

The definition of what the word signifies also changes when it is further defined as to what kind of budget is being discussed. *Personnel budget*, *capital budget*, and *operating budget* may all have different meanings to the same department head as to his or her ability to use the funds contained in each specific budget. These interpretations many times are the result of past experiences in being able or unable to use the funds that on paper have been approved by management. The supervisor who is aware of the multiplicity of interpretations possible by the receiver in decoding messages will be more effective when encoding a message to be transmitted.

Communication between line and staff personnel can be strained. This is often due to a failure of management to clearly define the duties, responsibilities, authority and reporting mechanism of each employee.

If management has elected to use staff employees in the traditional sense of support to line operations, then this should be made absolutely clear to both line and staff. However, if management has elected to use staff to function in a dual capacity with both support and line responsibility, then this should be made clear. Distinct lines of authority and responsibility will promote harmony and good communication between line and staff employees.

After reviewing the difficulties encountered during the process of communications and the steps for improvement, the supervisor is ready to practice the art of effective communication by making the following resolution: I will make each conversation a challenge for a new beginning, a pleasant course and a happy ending.

REFERENCES

1. Edwards, T., et al. *The New Dictionary of Thoughts*. Cincinnati, Ohio: Standard, 1977, p. 113.
2. Ibid., 636.
3. Ibid., 113.
4. Ibid., 112.
5. Ibid., 112.

Sexist language in health care facilities

> *Every vital development in language is a development of feeling as well.*
>
> —T.S. Eliot, *Philip Massinger*

John L. DiGaetani
Assistant Professor of English
Hofstra University
Hempstead, New York

AS MORE AND MORE women have left their homes to pursue careers, language has been changing to reflect the new social realities. While some of these changes seem a bit silly and may not last, others represent changes in the language of professional life that affect all health care facilities. In a field where thousands of women have achieved positions of power and responsibility, sensitivity to sexist language is especially important.

THE QUANDARY OF ADDRESS

When the new convention of addressing a woman as "Ms." was first introduced, it met with much derision and skepticism. Such criticisms were soon overcome, as the term filled a real need, permitting a graceful way around some otherwise awkward dilemmas. Some women object to being addressed with this new term, however. But Ms. is both logi-

Health Care Superv, 1984,3(1),48–52
© 1984 Aspen Publishers, Inc.

cal and neat, and many women in professional settings prefer it.

Another problem arises in writing to a company or a department without knowing the name of the person who will receive the letter. Here the best solution is simply to do some research and learn the full name of the intended recipient. When it is not possible to learn the particular name, other forms of address should be used, where appropriate. One option, used in writing to a committee or a board, is to address the letter to "Members of the Committee" or "Members of the Board" or "Members of the Department." Another possibility, if the recipient has a known title, is to use the title without a name (for example, "Dear Director," "Dear Manager," or "Dear Doctor").

THE MASCULINE SINGULAR PRONOUN

Other examples of sexism continue to exist in our daily language. One of these is the practice of using "he" whenever the writer finds it necessary to refer to a singular unspecified person. Another troublesome situation occurs when the gender of the pronoun reflects the assumed gender of its antecedent. For example, "Each doctor in the hospital is expected to submit his X11 report no later than the second Tuesday of each month," or "Each nurse should submit her Z23 report weekly."

The traditional rationale for using the masculine pronoun when the gender is unknown is that, in such cases, the masculine form is to be considered neutral. Or put another way, unless otherwise specified, the masculine pronoun can refer to either male or female. Grammarians and historians of the English language claim that the English word "man" is derived from the German word "mann," which refers to either sex. This is a knowledgeable and elegant rationale, but it does not change the fact that many people do see "man" as having a gender connotation.

One recent study found that when the pronouns he, his or him were used in a story (made up for purposes of the experiment by the investigators) that could have referred to either a male or a female, 65 percent of the people who read the story assumed that a male was intended. The subjects of this study were more than 500 college students (approximately half male and half female) who were no doubt familiar with the neutral-masculine rule, but who nevertheless—on the level of comprehension—often translated he into a male figure.[1]

If one is neither a budding psychologist nor a militant feminist, none of this may appear particularly important. But as a professional, one will likely be placed in situations where sensitivity to the issues of sexism, especially as it affects writing, will be important. Not only will one's sensitivity lead to word choices that can favorably impress readers and listeners who are themselves sensitive to the effects of sexism on language, but one will find also that a judicious delicacy in choosing language can prevent blundering into serious difficulties with affirmative action officers, legal advisers, union grievance officers and even the courts. In hospital administration the number of sexual harassment and sexual discrimination charges is already significant. Along with the charges have come victories, both in and out of court, by those who have claimed to have been discriminated against or sexually harassed on the job.

Most of these charges are brought by women, and the scope of sexual harassment cases heard by the courts has already included alleged instances of vulgar language and double entendres directed at women. So it is not farfetched to imagine that any administrative language that inflexibly adheres to the neutral-masculine pronoun rule is itself discriminatory. Psychological studies such as the one cited would support these charges despite the English language convention that prescribes the usage of masculine singular pronouns in references to both genders. Modern evidence overwhelms ancient practice, and overall the writer must agree that the world that language describes is largely a male world in which females are often relegated to lesser positions. But this is not the impression modern American health care facilities can afford to create. As a result, most documents intended for a public audience, such as advertising brochures or annual reports of publicly held hospitals, should be carefully written and edited to avoid any appearance of sexist language, including the repeated use of only the masculine singular pronoun.

SEXIST JOB TITLES

Aside from sexist pronouns, the problem of equal treatment is also complicated by sexist job titles, such as salesman, repairman, chairman and so on. Some of the attempts to create nonsexist titles have resulted in the creation of unnatural and cumbersome terms; however, the trend in hospital administration and government is toward using nonsexist titles whenever they do not sound silly. A repairman can easily become a repair person or repair staff in all official documents. And official documents can be used as evidence in court and elsewhere of the sexist or nonsexist climate within a medical facility. Charges of sex discrimination are weakened when a hospital or other health facility can show its commitment to nondiscriminatory practices,

---

Charges of sex discrimination are weakened when a hospital or other health facility can show its commitment to nondiscriminatory practices.

---

which may well begin with a consistent use of nonsexist language in official documents and correspondence.

Fortunately, in hospitals many of the job titles are already nonsexist, such as physician, nurse, orderly, and patient. Twenty years ago, physician automatically meant a male, and nurse automatically meant a female, but these sexual stereotypes have become less automatic because of changing social realities, and the terms themselves are not inherently sexist.

SOLUTIONS

Finding adequate substitutes for the masculine singular pronoun is not easy, and many proposed solutions sound graceless and awkward. These proposals come down to three possibilities: (1) using a masculine-feminine combination with a slash mark (he/she), (2) using both masculine and feminine pronouns wherever a third-person singular pronoun is needed, (3) replacing all unspecified gender references with plurals (their) or (4) rewriting the sentence to avoid pronouns.

The he/she option strikes many readers as jarring; it certainly fails the conversational test and rarely appears in print. The he-or-she option can become excessively wordy and cumbersome, especially when repeated frequently. On the other hand, the plural form, *their*, seems neither jarring nor cumbersome and is conversational, yet it can become awkward or excessively repetitious and does not always work.

Take, for example, the following illustration:

The policyholder should sign the claims form and mail it promptly to his agent.

Using the plural option, this becomes:

Policyholders should sign the claims form and mail it promptly to their agent.

Or perhaps it would be better this way:

Policyholders should sign the claims forms and mail them promptly to their agents.

Either revised version, though conversational, seems to suggest a crowded picture of masses signing forms, which was not the writer's intent.

Another option, which unfortunately does not always work, is rewriting the sentence to avoid pronouns altogether. For example:

The auditor for St. Francis Convalescent Home says that the bookkeeper there keeps his accounting books in very good order.

This becomes:

The auditor for St. Francis Convalescent Home says that the bookkeeper there keeps the accounting books in very good order.

By avoiding a pronoun altogether, the writer solves the problem quite easily; but this method will not always work because the writer sometimes needs a pronoun to make clear sense, and sometimes only a singular pronoun will do. For example:

Each orderly must ensure cleanliness in his ward.

This sentence can be changed to:

Each orderly must ensure cleanliness in the ward.

Or:

Orderlies must ensure cleanliness in their wards.

These changes can cause confusion, sacrificing clarity for gender neutrality.

Another more radical solution is to rewrite an entire sentence to avoid sexist language. This is sometimes necessary when other solutions simply will not work. For example:

A nurse should recognize her biases when dealing with minority patients.

This sentence can be rephrased as:

Bias should not influence nursing care.

Be cautious, however, with extensive rewriting to avoid sexist language. It is difficult to change a sentence so radically without altering its meaning, at least in a subtle way.

In summary, there is no easy, all-inclusive solution for the problems of sexist language. Fortunately there are many different solutions—such as the ones suggested here—so that in most, though not all, situations it is possible to find a graceful and acceptable way to avoid sexist language. In lengthy pieces of writing, such as long reports, occasional uses of a "he" or "him" will probably be unavoidable. If possible, the occasional use of "she" and "her" will help to get across the idea that an individual of either sex is being referred to.

Whatever the situation, it is wise to stay alert to the temper of the times and to the ideas of those people with whom one must deal. Reading and listening carefully are important here. And even then, one may occasionally make a false step—such as adopting the "he or she" solution only to discover that the boss regards this as a faddish affectation that he or she has no use for. As usual, what matters most is not knowing all things for all situations, but making sensible decisions about what does and does not work for the intended audience and the writer's situation.

REFERENCE

1. Moulton, J., Robinson, G.M., and Elias, C. "Sex Bias in Language Use." *American Psychologist* 33 (November 1978): 1032–36.

Part II
Ups and Downs in Organizational Communication

The supervisor's central role in organizational communication

Charles R. McConnell
Vice President for Employee Affairs
The Genesee Hospital
Rochester, New York

"THE TROUBLE with this place is there's no communication."

"I don't know what's going on around here. Nobody ever tells me anything."

"You mean we've both been trying to clean up the same problem for three weeks? Why didn't somebody tell me what was happening?"

Hardly a supervisor works who has not at one time or another made such statements or asked such questions or otherwise verbally condemned the general state of communication throughout the organization. Certainly these are fairly common remarks, and whether spoken in simple bewilderment or outright anger they reveal the speaker's frustrations with the problems encountered when information they need to help them do their jobs properly is unknown or unavailable to them.

Notice, however, where all of the

Health Care Superv, 1985,3(2),77–86
© 1985 Aspen Publishers, Inc.

opening quotations seem to place most of the blame for incomplete or nonexistent communication. The implication is that "I," the speaker, am communicating properly while the rest of the organization is not. The guilt seems to be laid on the biggest villain encountered in organizational life—the ever-blameful, never accountable, rarely identified "they." The usual implication is that "I" am clean but "they" are *not* communicating.

At times an individual may be fully justified in saying that the organization suffers from a general lack of communication. However, having said so one should then be willing to accept the possibility that a portion of this lack may be due to one's own position in the communication process. Communication, much like charity, begins at home, with each individual communicator. Thus it would perhaps be wise to examine one's own behavior to determine whether everything possible has been done to enhance communication.

THE FORMAL CHANNELS

Referring to Figure 1, imagine yourself as the individual supervisor in the block labeled YOU. As long as you are anywhere in the organization's management structure, this diagram will apply. For the first-line supervisor, the block for YOUR SUBORDINATES represents the members of the working group. For a manager working at a higher level

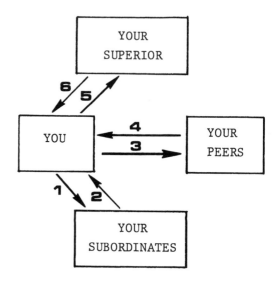

Figure 1. Formal channels of communication.

within the organization, this block may represent one, two or several lower-level supervisors.

The block labeled YOUR PEERS can be taken to represent other supervisors or managers, particularly those at or near your own level in the organization. The block labeled YOUR SUPERIOR can ordinarily be thought of as referring to a single person—the boss (although it is indeed possible for "the boss" to be several people such as a board of directors, if you happen to be a chief operating officer).

The six arrows in the figure represent the more or less formal channels along which people communicate. Information originating with you, the individual supervisor, flows outward to your boss, your peers and the employees in your work group. Likewise, information from those three people or groups flows back to you. These six channels represent the bulk of every supervisor's formal lines of communication, those built into the organization's structure and expected to exist in normal working relationships. Informal channels are more difficult to identify since they involve a person's friends, speaking acquaintances or work associates within the organization.

INFLUENCING INFORMATION FLOW

Speaking of the formal channels only, the three that lead away from you (numbers 1, 3 and 5) are completely controllable by you. It is solely up to the individual supervisor whether anything at all travels in any of these channels. To traverse one of these three channels a piece of information must originate with the supervisor and be transmitted to someone else through some effort on the part of the supervisor.

The supervisor can exert a relatively high degree of control over what comes back on channel number 2, the return channel from the employees; a moderate amount of influence over what comes back on channel number 4, from your peers; and even some influence on what comes back on channel number 6, from the boss. By far the most effective way to stimulate information flow through the incoming channels is to assure that the paths leading outward are open and operating.

By far the most effective way to stimulate information flow through the incoming channels is to assure that the paths leading outward are open and operating.

Subordinates

The easiest direction in which to begin working to improve one's communication is downward. Regarding the employees in the work group, formal relationships are weighted in favor of the supervisor. Subordinates rely on the supervisor for instructions, praise, criticism and information about their jobs and about the organization. Communication with your employees, as well as with anyone else in the organization, is first and foremost a matter of attitude and only second a matter of mechanics and performance.

There are at least three kinds of information you should pass along to the employees in your group: information that enables them to perform their jobs; information that helps instill in them the proper attitudes (since employee attitude is closely related to job performance); and the knowledge that they can come to you with questions and problems and find a ready listener. The primary task in communicating with your employees is to pass to them all the things they need in a way that necessitates or encourages feedback.

The conscientious practice of delegation can go a long way toward establishing sound communication from the employees to the supervisor. The establishment of reasonable deadlines for task completion and follow-up will stimulate feedback, as long as such deadlines are specific (not "as soon as you can" or "when you get a chance").

In applying deadlines, one should be reasonable or even a bit on the loose side if the situation permits. For example, imagine that it is Monday morning and the manager of food service discovers the need for a special quality report to be presented at a Friday morning staff meeting. The manager believes that the person to whom the compilation of the report should be assigned could reasonably be expected to have it done by Wednesday morning. If pushed, the employee could perhaps have the report done sometime on Tuesday. The manager gives the employee the reasonable deadline of 10 A.M. Wednesday knowing that the employee has plenty of time in which to respond. The manager wishes, if possible, to save the balance of Wednesday and all of Thursday as a cushion against the unexpected. However, if 10 A.M. Wednesday arrives and no report has reached the manager, what should then be done? The only choice open to the manager who wishes to have any chance of success in establishing information flow from the employees is to immediately get back to the delinquent employee.

Reasonable deadlines are but a small part of the process. The crucial step is prompt follow-up when a deadline is missed. It is easy enough to establish a deadline, but it is easier still to let it slide. Procrastination breeds procrastination; if you come across as a procrastinating boss, most of the employees in the group will quickly become attuned to this behavior, and many of them will behave the same way.

The example of the food service manager described an attempt to build into one's communications the essential two-way characteristic. The employee is given what is needed to do the job—the basic assignment. Further built into the assignment is the requirement to return to the supervisor that which is needed to be known—the feedback, or in this case the report itself.

However, not everything that should come to the supervisor from the employees can be mandated by organizational structure or controlled by assignments or deadlines. Some items originating solely with the employees must be brought to the supervisor's attention at the employees' initiative. Neither the organizational structure nor job descriptions require a clerk, for example, to tell a supervisor that he or she has been approached by a union organizer. Nothing guarantees that the supervisor will learn that two employees do not get along particularly well with each other. Such information will flow toward the supervisor only if the employees feel comfortable about such communication with the boss. The creation of the necessary atmosphere requires the supervisor to give the employee every opportunity to communicate. There are many pieces of helpful information that the supervisor will never know exist, let alone ever receive, unless he or she creates an atmosphere in which the employees are willing to provide the information.

The phrase "need to know" applies to far more than the information that is necessary for an employee to do a job. A side trip into the literature of employee motivation will reveal that fairly concrete, recognizable factors, such as descent wages and a comprehensive health insurance plan, are not quite the all-powerful, all-encompassing motivators they were once thought to be. Equally important are factors such as appreciation for work well-done, the feeling that one is a part of an organization rather than a mere cog in a wheel and a feeling that one is reasonably included in the life, activities and destiny of the organization.

Creation of a true communication climate requires sensitivity to the wants, needs and desires of the employees and at least a general knowledge of the practice of human relations. Although you cannot sense in advance what should be coming from the employees, you can nevertheless provide the opportunity and encouragement for them to speak up. In other words, the age-old claim that "My door is always open" should be more attitude than platitude.

Consider the example of Glenn, the manager of building services for a sizable medical center. Glenn had achieved a true open-door policy as a matter of successful practice, and thus he was able to learn, through one of his housekeeping employees, that a number of people in the department were upset and complaining vehemently because they had heard they were going to lose out on an expected holiday. For several years in a row the organization had declared the Friday after Thanksgiving a paid holiday, though in fact it was not one of the paid holidays listed in the employee manual. Strong rumor claimed that the medical center was experiencing a bad year under the new reimbursement structure and that the current position would not permit the luxury of an additional paid holiday. Glenn himself had not heard the story, and had he not been a manager who encouraged input from his staff he might never have learned of the unhappiness of some of his employees.

Glenn's first reaction was to admit he knew nothing about the story and promise to take steps to find out the truth. He approached the vice president for personnel services, who acknowledged that under prevailing conditions the personnel office had considered not granting the holiday, but added that they had recently decided to declare the extra holiday as usual. Together Glenn and the vice president were able to determine that the story probably started through speculative talk by some of the personnel clerks who had overheard privileged information. Since a decision had been made, Glenn urged the vice president to release the holiday declaration a few days earlier than planned and immediately reported back to his employees that the rumor was untrue and the holiday would be declared. In doing so, he managed to ease the doubts of a number of people, and in the process he removed a troublesome factor that could have significantly affected his employees' performance.

Peers

Not quite as easy to deal with as communication from your employees is the stimulation of feedback from your peers. In this case you have no organizational clout; in fact there may be no organizational policy whatsoever requiring supervisors and managers to keep each other informed.

In this matter of lateral communication it is important to stimulate information flow on the incoming channels by assuring that the outgoing channels are open and in active use. The "golden rule" approach is clearly the most effective: strive to keep others informed as you would like to be kept informed. However, communication with other members of management is not nearly as controllable as communication with your own employees. Your degree of success will depend largely on the attitudes of those in the upper levels of the organization. For that matter, if all members of management try to communicate as much as you may be trying, then problems are minimized. However, if you must report to a non-

communicative superior who does little to stimulate interaction between subordinate supervisors, the task is then difficult indeed.

Success in lateral communication depends on the degree to which you consider the other person and remember him or her as you would wish to be remembered. First and simplest, you should make sure you are available to others. Supervisors may complain about seemingly endless meetings, but regardless of whether the information received in such meetings is valuable, the meetings themselves nevertheless have value in that they place supervisors in proximity to other members of management. The supervisor who is asked to report on what is happening in the department may seem to have little of immediate relevance to say to others; however, an item offered in the way of general information may prove unexpectedly useful to someone who hears it.

Do not overlook the value of lunch time and coffee breaks. If you are in the habit of eating alone at your desk or skipping coffee breaks, you are missing some of the best potential communication opportunities. A great deal of useful information flows in the informal settings of lunch time and the coffee break.

"Don't say it, write it," reads the heading on the standard little note pad available by the thousands. "Avoid oral orders," says the similar action-request pad used by large numbers of organizations. Once the supervisor has put something in writing, he or she must next consider who in addition to the direct addressee should receive a copy.

The "need-to-know" rationale may be stretched somewhat in relation to many of your peers. At least the benefit of the doubt should be extended regarding the intensity of the need. For instance, although you may not absolutely need a given piece of information to enable you to continue doing your job, you may nevertheless "need" this information to enable you to fully understand a situation or to add to your knowledge of what is happening in the rest of the organization.

There is no effort wasted in remembering someone now and then with a courtesy copy of a letter or memorandum even though the subject may not seem immediately relevant to him or her. Unless proprietary information is involved, the criterion need not always be whether the person needs to know. Rather, you may ask who should *not* be included in the distribution because they clearly cannot use the information in any way, shape or form. In other words, if in doubt, include the person. The extra copy provided out of courtesy is virtually insignificant in cost, and a bargain if it clarifies another supervisor's understanding of a situation, avoids an incorrect reaction or stops rumor before it starts.

For example, a medical center that counted among its employees some two dozen senior managers recognized the need to assure thorough lateral communication among them.

They experimented with the idea of sending copies of all communications to everyone but immediately dropped this approach when the difficulty of distributing 24 copies of every memo was encountered. Instead, management adopted the idea of the reading file. This file includes a copy of every letter and memo written by all 24 of the senior managers in a day. One secretary is responsible for assembling the reading file each day. The day's file is circulated, and each recipient is expected to pass it along within one working day of the time it is received. Each reader can, as he or she chooses, skim the bulk of the file and concentrate on items of particular interest. The fact that it sometimes takes a few days for the file to work its way through the entire group appears to produce no significant problem. The reading file has helped create the feeling that people are going out of their way to keep each other informed about what is happening.

Another way to stimulate communication from your peers is by using forms such as the standard reply memo. This is a three-part form with interleaved carbon. There is a space for entering a handwritten message; you then snap off and retain the last part of the three-part set as a record copy. The recipient has a space in which to enter a reply, and having done so will retain the second part of the set and return the first part—including both message and reply—to the sender. This is of particular value in eliciting responses to specific questions, and it is also representative of an attitude that should characterize everyone's approach to communication in the working world: make it as easy as possible for the person from whom information is desired to provide it.

Superiors

The communication channel from the boss back to the supervisor can be the most difficult one to open because it is the one over which the individual exercises the least influence.

The communication channel from the boss back to the supervisor can be the most difficult one to open because it is the one over which the individual exercises the least influence.

If the superior is a communicator who tries as hard as the supervisor, there may be little problem. In fact, the problem would be even less than that of getting information from peers and subordinates, since organizational structure, tradition and general practice all favor the downward flow of information.

Should you feel, however, that you have difficulty getting information from the boss, perhaps the place to start is with an examination of your own attitude and availability. Your view of yourself may easily hamper your appreciation of how you may be viewed by your immediate superior.

You must step back and view yourself in action from the boss' perspective. Does your interest seem to be confined to your own department and generally to your own immediate sphere of activity, or do you come across as being generally interested in the total organization and its objectives? Do you always appear to be open to communication even though you may confront information you do not want to hear? That is, are you willing to take in and assess *all* information that comes your way?

Admittedly, matters of attitude can be subtle. Availability, however, is an entirely different matter. The boss should be able to reach the supervisor whenever he or she has something that must be communicated. The supervisor whose communication posture is passive—who takes no initiative, seeming to sit back and wait for the boss to initiate all communication—has perhaps forgotten that he or she represents only one of numerous contact points with which the boss must stay in touch.

At times it may seem as though the boss is an extremely difficult person to reach. If this is the case, you might improve communication by first looking for patterns in the boss's availability. Is this person most likely to be in the office first thing in the morning? Last thing in the afternoon? Perhaps for a brief period immediately following lunch? Insofar as possible, you might consider adjusting your own availability so as to be on hand when the boss is on hand.

Also, there are some positive steps

you can take to stimulate communication from the boss. Depending on the individual boss, however, these steps may have to be taken gently and diplomatically. Just as you should never procrastinate on a deadline given to an employee, neither should you allow the boss to procrastinate on a deadline he or she has handed down. If the boss has assigned a deadline, whether oral or written, respect the deadline and respond by the designated time even if the task is not complete or the boss has made no move to initiate follow-up. You should make it a practice never to let a deadline go by without some kind of positive response, even if you are certain that the boss would let it slide.

Here again the three-part message form can be extremely useful in getting responses to direct questions. Brief, specific questions requiring short answers encourage return communication by making it easy to communicate. For example, the director of personnel development and training for an association of hospitals was interested in the status of a proposal to provide shared educational services for members. The director had difficulty securing an audience with the boss, the association's vice president, because of the latter's hectic schedule. They were constantly missing each other. The director of personnel development and training condensed her current need to three concise questions as follows:

Regarding the shared education proposal
1. *Do you agree with it as written?*

2. *Will it be presented at the next board meeting?*
3. *Do you need any more input from me before then?*

She left this message in the most obvious place—taped to the receiver of the vice president's telephone. Later on the same day she discovered, on returning from a meeting, that the vice president had been in and gone out again, but had found time to answer her questions. The reply portion of the message form read:

1. *Yep.*
2. *Yep.*
3. *Nope.*

This example also partly addresses the notion of completed staff work. Usually the boss wants to communicate with all directly reporting supervisors, but often the boss is also a fairly busy person. Many higher managers do not want supervisors bringing them problems; most successful top managers look for answers rather than questions for which they are expected to provide answers.

If you expect complete and open communication with the boss, you should not go to that superior with only problems and questions. When a problem exists, first analyze the difficulty, look at it from every conceivable angle, come up with several alternatives, and sort the alternatives down to the ones that appear most practical and workable. When you go to the boss you should be able to say something like, "Here is a problem. Here is why it is a problem. Here is what I would like to do, and here is what I require from you to be able to do so. Do you agree or disagree?"

All of these suggestions may work with your boss. However, it is equally possible that none of them will work. It depends entirely on the individual boss, his or her approach to communication and the relationship that you have established. If your superior is an apparent noncommunicator who seems to avoid you, you can sit back and complain about how "There's no communication around this place." Or you can try some of the techniques that have been suggested here. Even if you manage to open up communication only slightly through one or two of the channels, this level of communication will still be more than existed before.

THE KEY IS YOU

The supervisor's position in organizational communication may be compared to that of a two-way radio. If the supervisor—that is, the radio—wishes to receive, you must first ensure that the set is transmitting loud and clear on all frequencies so that others will know you have the capability to receive. You must then also be aware of all other senders' frequencies and be able to fine-tune your equipment to them (that is, be aware of their availability, their needs and the way they work) and keep the channels open.

The process of communication involves the transfer of meaning. The tools of communication—visual symbols, audible symbols, motions and so on—are at best weak devices for transferring meaning. They are effective tools only when communication is regarded as a two-way street on which heavy traffic must flow in both directions.

The desire for two-way communication may seem noble and "only fair." However, there is a trap in the very notion of fairness or equal effort. Clearly, the best way to stimulate information flow through your incoming channels is to make certain that your outgoing channels are open and actively working. This action does not guarantee, however, that your best efforts at improving communication will always be reciprocated. You may find that it is ultimately necessary to go more than halfway more than half of the time and fully expect that some of your consideration of others will never be repaid in kind. If you feel you are stuck with the short end of the stick, ask yourself one simple question: "Who is the primary beneficiary of my improved communication?" Everything you do to keep the communication channels open and to ensure that others are remembered ultimately benefits your own communication.

Perhaps the next time you hear about a lack of communication, it may be that there is precisely that, no communication, not even from the complainer.

On the grapevine

George D. Pozgar
Administrator
St. John's Episcopal Hospital
Smithtown, New York

"Where no wood is, *there* the fire goeth out: so where *there is* no talebearer, the strife ceaseth" (Prov. 26:20).

WHERE DID YOU hear it? *On the grapevine. I just found out. I don't want to be involved in this one. Don't tell anyone I told you so. I'll deny it if you say anything.* Sound familiar?

What is it that travels faster than the speed of light and is more powerful than a locomotive? Could it be the grapevine of rumors, rumblings, gossip, and shoptalk? The grapevine is generally referred to as informal and spontaneous communications built around social relationships in which everyone participates in the exchange of either social or business information. Each of us is usually a member of one or more social groups through which information is shared in an organization. In *Human Behavior at Work*, Keith Davis notes, "The informal grapevine coexists with

Health Care Superv, 1986,4(2),39–49
© 1986 Aspen Publishers, Inc.

management's formal communication system. The term 'grapevine' arose during the War Between the States. Intelligence telegraph lines were strung loosely from tree to tree in the manner of a grapevine. Since messages from the lines often were incorrect or confusing, any rumor was said to be from the grapevine."[1]

The grapevine will often take over when there is a breakdown in the formal organization. Employees are likely to depend on information obtained from the informal organization even though it is often viewed as being somewhat misleading and unreliable. Employees and supervisors alike get entangled in the grapevine because of information gaps. The motivating forces behind an active grapevine include the need for job security, the desire to draw attention to or away from oneself, the need for companionship, the need to share mutual concerns, and the desire to give the appearance of being in the know or to advance one's personal aims.

Whether it carries small talk or an important and intriguing conversation, the grapevine is a form of communication. According to Koontz and O'Donnell, the grapevine ". . . thrives on information not openly available to the entire group, whether because it is regarded as confidential, because formal lines of communication are inadequate to disperse it, or because it is of the kind that would never be formally disclosed. Even a management that conscientiously informs employees through company bulletins or newspapers never so completely or expeditiously discloses all information of interest as to make the grapevine purposeless."[2]

GRAPEVINE POLITICS

Rumors and hearsay are the propagators of war, and their snowball effect has been the downfall of cities. "By the blessing of the upright the city is exalted: but it is overthrown by the mouth of the wicked."[3] Even ancient kings used the power of the tongue for political gain. "The Great King grew alarmed, and after his manner undertook a diplomatic diversion. An agent primed with fifty gold talents was sent over to Greece with orders to stir up trouble among Sparta's neighbors at home. Thebes fell to the bait and declared war against her one-time ally."[4] Even in the modern world, so-called press leaks are used for political gain or as a method of revenge by disgruntled persons. Managers sometimes distribute information through planned leaks or judiciously placed "just-between-you-and-me" remarks.[5]

Supervisors must be careful not to depend on the grapevine as their only source of information. As noted, the grapevine's validity and reliability are questionable. Because of poor memories and inaccurate perceptions, truth is often distorted, leading to false conclusions and bad decisions. "Calumny is like the wasp that worries you, which it is not best to try to get rid of unless you are sure of

> *Although the supervisor must not overestimate the importance of the grapevine, it is equally important that he or she not underestimate its value. After all, it often focuses on a problem, and it is a means of communication.*

slaying it; for otherwise it returns to the charge, more furious than ever."[6]

THE GRAPEVINE AS A BAROMETER

Although the supervisor must not overestimate the importance of the grapevine, it is equally important that he or she not underestimate its value. After all, it often focuses on a problem, and it is a means of communication. It is a barometer of public opinion, attitudes, and organizational concerns. It has the capability of carrying information that is both helpful and detrimental to the organization.

Every supervisor should ask, "Does the formal organization meet the informational needs of employees?" If not, a more effective use of the formal lines of communication should be developed. In *Management,* James Stoner declares that "the grapevine in organizations is made up of several informal communication networks that overlap and intersect at a number of points; that is, some well-informed individuals are likely to belong to more than one informal network. Grapevines show admirable disregard for rank or authority and may link organization members in any combination of directions—horizontal, vertical and diagonal."[7]

The grapevine is an extremely intricate communications network. The combinations of up, down, and across information linkages are practically infinite. As pointed out previously, depending on the perceived relative importance of the information being transmitted, some of it will be short-lived whereas other bits will build and travel through the network in countless combinations.

The best-kept secret does not exist—if you know it, its secrecy is most likely not secure. The following cases illustrate how information can travel and be distorted in the organization.

Vandalism in the parking lot

Jane Doe, a technician in the department of radiology, suggested, while eating lunch with four of her friends, that John Smith, a dietary aide, might be one of several persons responsible for vandalism in the employee parking lot. By the end of the day Smith was approached by his department head regarding the rumors. Smith denied the accusations. The diagram in Figure 1 illustrates, somewhat simplistically, how this rumor traveled through the informal organization.

Doe's remarks, whether true or not, were devastating to Smith's character and integrity. The real culprits were caught several days later, and Smith

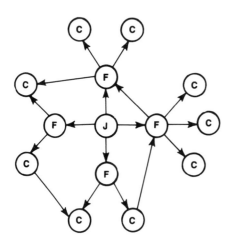

Figure 1. Illustration of how a rumor travels through the informal organization. J = Jane Doe; F = friends of Jane Doe; C = coworkers with Jane Doe's friends.

was not one of them. The distrust and quick judgment of fellow employees caused Smith to eventually resign and seek employment elsewhere. This case illustrates the difficulties encountered and the traumatic effect the informal organization can have on a fellow employee.

The ten-minute rumor

Fred Jones, a department head, read a want ad in the local newspaper for an assistant controller. The ad specified that resumés for the position should be returned to 400 Main Street, the same street address as corporate headquarters. Jones logically assumed that the advertisement was for the replacement of the assistant controller. He reported this information to his supervisor, an assistant administrator, who in turn discussed it with the administrator. The control-

ler was somewhat surprised to learn of the ad from the administrator. The information was passed on to the assistant controller who reacted somewhat lightheartedly but with concern. The diagram in Figure 2 illustrates the flow of information through the formal organization.

The want ad was reviewed and it was determined that a personnel recruiting agency, having the same address as corporate headquarters, placed the ad. Thus the rumor was short-lived when the correct information was promptly disseminated back down the formal organization. Failure to correct the rumor could have resulted in its further spread on the grapevine. This case illustrates the flow of information both upward and downward in the formal organization.

The potential for distorted communication in the formal organization increases with corporate size and the resulting interjection of additional hi-

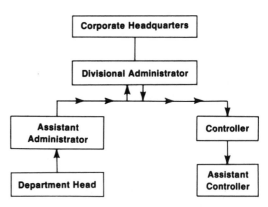

Figure 2. Illustration of how information is properly disseminated through the formal organization.

erarchical levels into the corporate structure. Information becomes more difficult to obtain, and the first-line supervisor becomes increasingly frustrated; out of necessity he or she must depend on the less reliable informal grapevine for information.

The theory of cognitive dissonance

. . . states the much observed phenomenon that recipients of information unconsciously focus on and relay only the information that reinforces their preexisting attitudes, while filtering out conflicting information. To the extent that adverse information conflicts with the recipient's basic attitudes by showing failure, it [the information] is particularly subject to this unconscious filtering. Even absent the distorting impact of preexisting attitudes on information flow, experimental evidence suggests that serial relay of information results in significant information loss. Information theorists have formulated the rule that each additional relay in a communications system halves the message while doubling the "noise" and only a very diluted message will reach the top through regular lines of communication.[8]

A LEGAL PERSPECTIVE

The inappropriate use of the grapevine can give rise to slander suits. Even though the courts are relatively skeptical about hearsay and for the most part will not allow it to be accepted as evidence, there are more than twenty exceptions under which it can be accepted. In the following four instances, certain words are slanderous per se, meaning that damage is presumed without proof thereof and should be considered gossip's forbidden zone:

1. words imputing a crime to the plaintiff;
2. words imputing to the plaintiff a loathsome and communicable disease that banishes him or her from society (usually limited to venereal disease);
3. words affecting the plaintiff in his or her trade or profession, such as calling a physician a "quack"[9] or a nurse "inept"; and
4. in some jurisdictions, words imputing unchastity to a person.

Grapevine gossip can infringe on one's right to privacy. Such invasion can be injurious to one's reputation, causing substantial emotional distress which can lead to a slander suit and result in monetary damages being awarded to the slandered party. The basic purpose of a defamation action is to vindicate a person's good name.

A good reputation is an aid, and a bad reputation is a deterrent in obtaining almost any kind of lawful employment. This aspect of the interest in reputation is primarily a property interest, a thing of monetary value. On the other hand, the interest in reputation may be considered to be an interest involving personality and human dignity. The fact that long settled law permits a substantial award for damages in many actions for defamation in which there is no evidence of any monetary loss to the plaintiff makes this clear.[10]

The grapevine is responsible for countless character assassinations.

"The calumniator (or contemptuous person) inflicts wrong by slandering the absent; and he who gives credit to the calumny (a false and malicious statement designed to injure someone's reputation) before he knows it is true, is equally guilty. The person traduced is doubly injured, by him who propagates, and by him who credits the slander."[11]

Words have the power to condemn or to vindicate. In 1535 Sir Thomas More was beheaded for offering an opinion to King Henry VIII regarding a matrimonial problem. Sir Walter Raleigh was accused of treason and sentenced to death in 1603. His death penalty was commuted to imprisonment. The case against him was based on hearsay and unsupported accusations that today would not stand up as sufficient evidence to convict him.

Rumors that certain residents of the Massachusetts Bay Colony were witches led to hundreds of arrests and a number of hangings. One resident of the colony was whipped and had his ears cut off for speaking loosely about the colony's government and church at Salem.[12] Fanatics, by slicing the thin edge of truth and reason, have often been responsible for the downfall of many innocent people.

It is of interest that the U.S. Supreme Court in *Nebraska Press Association v. Stuart, Judge, et al.* noted

. . . the events disclosed by the record took place in a community of 850 people. It is reasonable to assume that, without any news accounts being reprinted or broadcast, rumors would travel swiftly by word of mouth. One can only speculate on the accuracy of such reports, given the generative propensities of rumors; they could well be more damaging than reasonably accurate news accounts. But plainly a whole community cannot be restrained from discussing a subject intimately affecting life within it.[13]

NEGATIVE PROGRAMMING

We are not given much to cheer about. For the most part we are constantly flooded with negative information. The following topics illustrate a sampling of what can be presented by the media on a single Sunday afternoon:

The Newspaper
- "Eavesdropping on the Mob"
- "Study Links Exercise to Aging"
- "34 Americans Hurt in Blast in Greek Bar"
- "Elderly Woman Beaten"
- "Bicyclist Dies in Hit-and-Run"
- "Two Hurt in Separate Stabbings"

The Television
- *The Amazing Spiderman*
- *Jaws 3-D*
- *The Beast Must Die*
- *MAD*
- *Coma*

Local Theaters
- *The Killing Fields*
- *Runaway*
- *The Texas Chain Saw Massacre*
- *Tuff Turf*

When Monday morning arrives, the manager must:
- determine the impact of a Medicare freeze;

- reduce staffing and cut expenditures for supplies;
- implement right-to-know toxic waste regulations;
- prepare for a Joint Commission on the Accreditation of Hospitals survey;
- review the monthly budget with the supervisory manager;
- counsel an employee; and
- complete several employee evaluations.

The Amazing Spiderman may sound harmless, but its effect on the mind of a young child cannot be discounted. The news media—theater, radio, and TV—have bombarded society with negatives. It is little wonder that we are a negative generation. We rush to work, we rush home, we rush through our meals of fast food, and we rush through the newspaper with all of its annoying ads and horror stories. We watch "the box" and all of its soap operas, and we rush to bed and then wonder why our dreams are bad and why we always seem to be running from something. We need no psychoanalyst to tell us why we are more tired when we get up than when we go to bed.

The news at work is not always bleak, but we have been conditioned to pass on the sensational—after all, who wants to listen to anything less? Our grapevine conversations have been molded and programmed by the media to produce ills, not cures.

THE GOOD NEWS

But what about the good news and who is telling that story? Good news can also provide sensational grapevine talk. For example, it is comforting to know that we have, for the most part, been secure from the ravages of smallpox, yellow fever, cholera, and a host of other exotic diseases. Our fears are not the scourge of leprosy nor the worries of being bitten by an Anopheles mosquito and contracting malaria. We are not afflicted by the numerous diseases that are associated with malnutrition and suffered by many in third world countries such as Kenya, Tanzania, Pakistan, India, and Bangladesh.

The American system of health care, with all of its faults, remains the best in the world. In 1900 only 29 percent of Americans lived past the age of 75. Today, 40 percent do so. In 1900 we reached middle age in our 20s; today it is in our late 30s.[14] In less than a century we have given ourselves the most precious gift of all—time. This is good news. As a matter of fact, it is sensational news, and few of us are aware of it. A more positive grapevine can be developed by exposing ourselves to the good news at home, work, and play.

DEVELOPING A POSITIVE GRAPEVINE

There is no magic button or technological gimmick that will resolve all the ailments of the grapevine. Management must develop a strategy for effectively communicating with supervisors and employees on a continuing basis. Communication is an ongoing process and not a one-time campaign.

---

*Management must develop a
strategy for effectively
communicating with supervisors
and employees on a continuing
basis. Communication is an
ongoing process and not a
one-time campaign.*

Supervisors will quickly find that where there is no news the grapevine will quickly create its own. Employees are more likely to speculate and spread rumors as to what is happening when management fails to communicate. Several vehicles for the dissemination of information will help in the development of a more healthy and positive grapevine.

- Use the grapevine to quickly distribute information. "Formal communication needs to come along to stamp 'official' on the news and to put it 'on the record,' which the grapevine cannot suitably do."[15]
- Create job descriptions that are current and that effectively present each employee's responsibilities. Understanding the importance of one's role in the organization translates into positive attitudes and feelings of self-worth.
- Provide employee orientation programs for new employees—to present the institution's mission, the employee's contribution to that mission, employee benefits, and so on. This can be accom-

plished with the aid of filmstrips, slides, and motion pictures.
- Publish employee handbooks describing hospital policies and personnel benefits, providing these to employees at the time of employment. Because employee benefits often change in the health care industry, it is important to distribute periodic updates.
- Disseminate information and hold departmental meetings to reveal employee concerns, clear up misunderstandings, and help in developing employee trust.
- Use employee newsletters, direct mail memorandums, and payroll inserts regarding social events, personnel benefit changes, and so forth; use bulletin boards for current information; and provide annual reports to employees.
- Use the employee evaluation, admittedly requiring much hard work, to enhance the relationship between employee and supervisor.
- Develop in-hospital supervisory training programs. If conscientiously pursued, these will ensure that supervisory managers have the opportunity to continually improve their communications skills.
- Keep supervisory managers fully informed so they do not become the source of misinformation. ". . . Management cannot communicate to workers unless management itself is informed. Not

only must management know (that is, be informed) but it must understand the information well enough to interpret it to others. Top management often fails to recognize this simple fact."[16] If the manager's door is open, there will be no guessing as to what is going on. Information will not be disseminated and false information will not be corrected if the door is closed. Face-to-face communication with employees is generally more effective than any other means of communication.

EMPLOYEE COMMITMENT THROUGH PARTICIPATION

Each employee becomes a more constructive contributor to the organization when he or she participates in the decision-making process. Employees should be encouraged to participate in the planning of social events as well as of business activities (e.g., employee picnics, annual Christmas party, fund-raising activities, and employee health programs).

. . . It would appear evident that if the organization expects its members to be committed, flexible, and in good communication with one another for the sake of overall organizational effectiveness, it is in effect asking them to be morally involved in the enterprise, to be committed to organizational goals, and to value these. And if it expects them to be involved to this degree, the organization must for its part provide rewards and conditions consistent with such involvement. It cannot merely pay more money to obtain commitment, creativity, and

flexibility; there must be the possibility of obtaining non-economic rewards such as autonomy, genuine responsibility, opportunities for challenge and for psychological growth.[17]

Managers can indirectly encourage employee participation in decision making by indicating a genuine interest in employee problems. Such interest becomes evident when managers do the following things:

- Provide career counseling. Employees who seemingly reach dead ends in their careers can many times be the most disgruntled. Career counseling services will demonstrate management's concern and desire to help guide each employee.
- Provide opportunities for job advancement through the active practice of promotion from within the organization.
- Use an employee suggestion program to reveal concerns of employees in the organization and provide management the opportunity to address employee concerns.

Overall, positive communication requires a healthy mix between the formal and informal environment of an organization. According to Keith Davis, a healthy organization has both a grapevine and official channels of communication. When both channels are working effectively, he states, they are somewhat of a complement to each other. Each (channel), he says, carries information particularly suited to its needs and capabilities so that together the two systems build effective communication in an organization.[18]

These are simple suggestions that will help in the development of a more positive grapevine. Supervisors cannot stop its use or control it, but they can help to direct it. An analysis of why, when, and where the communication gaps exist will enable managers to take appropriate steps toward the development of a healthy grapevine.

Managers have the ability to shape a grapevine that works with them, not against them. Improved contributions can be made to this grapevine. The following four-way test of self-questioning of managerial ideas, discussions, and actions, used by Rotary International, a service organization in Evanston, Illinois, suggests how to assess the information being transmitted:

1. Is it the truth?
2. Is it fair to all concerned?
3. Will it build good will and better friendships?
4. Will it be beneficial to all concerned?

•   •   •

It has been said that you reap what you sow. There are both sour and sweet grapes on every vine. There are grapes that have sweetened as they ripen and others that will always remain sour; both come from the same vineyard and many times from the same vine. The vintager must nurture the vineyard. The sunshine cannot be controlled, but pruning, watering, and fertilizing can. A healthy grapevine can produce a good harvest. Yet, just as the sunshine cannot be controlled, neither can the minds of employees. They can be provided with the necessary information and incentives to do their jobs. However, the manager has not failed if some remain sour. The interconnections and links of the grapevine are too complex for managers to expect or be expected to have an unblemished harvest. The sour will help bring about a deeper appreciation for the sweet.

Managers should not be discouraged when at harvest time after much labor, some sour grapes inevitably appear. Every grapevine has its sweet and sour—at best some grapes will always be average.

REFERENCES

1. Davis, K. *Human Behavior at Work*. New York: McGraw-Hill, 1977, p. 278.
2. Koontz, H., and O'Donnell, C. *Essentials of Management*. New York: McGraw-Hill, 1974, p. 231.
3. Prov. 11:11.
4. Robinson, C.E. *Hellas*. Boston: Beacon Press, 1955, p. 153.
5. Stoner, J.A.F. *Management*. Englewood Cliffs, N.J.: Prentice-Hall, 1982, p. 511.
6. Edwards, T., et al. *The New Dictionary of Thoughts*. Cincinnati: Standard, 1977, p. 72.
7. Stoner, *Management*, 511.
8. Solomon, L.D., Stevenson, R.B., Jr., and Schwartz, D.E. *Corporations*. St. Paul, Minn.: West Publishing, 1982, p. 794.
9. White v. Carroll, 42 N.Y. 161, 164 (1870).
10. Eldredge, L.H. *The Law of Defamation*. Indianapolis, Ind.: Bobbs-Merrill, 1978, p. 2.

11. Edwards, *The New Dictionary of Thoughts*, 72.

12. Wormeser, R.A. *The Story of the Law*. New York: Simon & Schuster, 1962, p. 309.

13. Nebraska Press Ass'n v. Stuart, Judge, et al., 427 U.S. 539 (1976).

14. Hayslick, L. "The Aging of Humans in the Cultured Cells." *Resident & Staff Physician* 30, no. 8 (1984): 37.

15. Davis, K. "Management Communication and the Grapevine." *Harvard Business Review* 31, no. 5 (1954): 45.

16. Davis, K. "Communication within Management." *Personnel* 31, no. 3 (1954): 213.

17. Schein, E.H. *Organizational Psychology*. Englewood Cliffs, N.J.: Prentice-Hall, 1965, p. 104.

18. Davis, K. "Grapevine Communication among Lower and Middle Managers." *Personnel Journal* 48, no. 4 (1969): 269.

Health care supervisors identify communication barriers in their supervisor–subordinate relationships

Steven Golen
Associate Professor

Robert Boissoneau
Professor
College of Business
Arizona State University
Tempe, Arizona

IN THE HEALTH care industry as in all other industries, the major ingredient for an efficient and productive organization is effective communication. Health care supervisors who possess effective interpersonal communication skills are generally perceived by their subordinates as being concerned about the human element involved in the organization. Thus, maintaining effective supervisor–subordinate relations is extremely important to improving job performance.

To foster this important relationship, health care supervisors need the ability to identify and to be aware of potential communication problems that may arise in this relationship. Once potential problems have been identified, then the supervisors will be able to handle these communication problems more effectively when they do occur. This article examines

Health Care Superv, 1987, 6(1), 26–38
© 1987 Aspen Publishers, Inc.

the barriers to effective communication that were perceived as most serious by health care supervisors in their supervisor–subordinate relationships.

RESEARCH PROCEDURES

Eighty-four health care supervisors who attended a supervisory training session at a major state university responded to a questionnaire. There were two parts to the questionnaire. The first part requested specific demographic information about the respondents. The second part instructed the respondents to indicate the seriousness of 32 potential barriers to effective communication based on their supervisor–subordinate relationships. The seriousness of these barriers was measured on a five-point scale from one signifying "not serious" to five signifying "very serious."

RESPONDENT CHARACTERISTICS

Age and sex profile
Thirty-nine percent of the respondents were between the ages of 31 and 40; 30 percent between 21 and 30; 23 percent between 41 and 50; and 8 percent were over 50. Sixty-three percent of the health care supervisors were females and 37 percent were males.

Type of health care organization
Fifty-one percent of the respondents were employed in private health care organizations and 49 percent were employed in public organizations.

Level of management
Fifty-nine percent of the personnel were in middle management; 21 percent were in upper management; and 20 percent were in lower management.

Years in position
Twenty-eight percent of the respondents had been in their present positions for less than 1 year; 46 percent from 1 to 5 years; 19 percent from 6 to 10 years; 5 percent from 11 to 15 years; and 2 percent from 16 to 20 years.

Number of employees supervised
Forty-two percent supervised more than 20 employees; 35 percent supervised 11 to 20 employees; and 23 percent supervised from 1 to 10 employees.

ANALYSIS AND DISCUSSION

The 32 communication barriers were ranked based on means. Table 1 includes the means for all the barriers. The five most serious barriers were perceived to be resistance to change, tendency not to listen, lack of feedback, having too many intermediate receivers between the sender and the intended receiver of information, and lack of trust. A discussion of all 32 barriers follows.

Table 1. Mean ratings and composite rank: Supervisor–subordinate relationship

Rank	Communication barrier	Mean
1	Resistance to change	4.21
2	Tendency not to listen	4.19
3	Lack of feedback	3.98
4	Too many gatekeepers	3.88
5	Lack of trust	3.87
6	Either-or thinking	3.82
7	Defensiveness	3.81
8	Hostile attitude	3.79
9	Know-it-all attitude	3.69
10	Emotional reactions	3.67
11	Prejudice or bias	3.66
12	Lack of credibility	3.60
13	Fear of distortion or omission of information	3.56
14	Lack of interest in the subject matter	3.56
15	Personality conflicts	3.55
16	Differences in perception	3.55
17	Prematurely jumping to conclusions	3.53
18	Physical noise and distractions	3.52
19	Overload or too much information	3.46
20	Poor organization of ideas	3.44
21	Poor timing of the message	3.28
22	Lack of understanding of technical language	3.25
23	Informal social groups or cliques	3.22
24	Use of profanity	3.14
25	Physical distance between sender and receiver of information	3.13
26	Overly competitive attitude	3.08
27	Status or position	3.07
28	Poor spatial arrangements	3.03
29	Inability to understand nonverbal communication	3.03
30	Speaking too loudly	2.73
31	Lack of health care knowledge	2.60
32	Inappropriate physical appearance	2.52

Resistance to change

In any health care organization supervisors must constantly change to meet the varying needs of the organization and its employees. Supervisors must be extremely cautious of how change affects their employees. Frequently, changes are met with employee resistance because these changes threaten to disrupt the employees' routine behaviors. The su-pervisors should communicate the changes positively in order to reduce employee anxiety. Supervisors need to explain clearly why the changes were made and how the changes are going to affect the employees individually.

Tendency not to listen

Poor listening skills have been cited as a major communication bar-

> *Poor listening skills have been cited as a major communication barrier across several professions; the health care industry is no exception.*

rier across several professions; the health care industry is no exception. Supervisors need to listen attentively, carefully, objectively, and empathetically to their employees. Supervisors must listen to understand and develop a climate that encourages employees to be open with their feelings. Effective supervisors can never listen too much.

Lack of feedback

For supervisors to understand whether they are meeting the needs of their employees, they must receive feedback from employees. Also, supervisors need to know whether their messages are understood completely by employees. Questioning the employees with sincerity about their understanding of a message helps promote effective communication. Supervisors must develop a policy that encourages and supports good employee communication.

Too many gatekeepers

Generally, the more transfer stations or gatekeepers between the subordinate and supervisor, the more likely the information can become distorted. Obviously, the supervisor needs to reduce the number of gate-keepers. If multiple channels must be followed for the sake of the chain of command, then the message should be as explicit as possible. Messages sent orally should be followed by written messages to ensure preservation of content throughout the channelling process. Also, supervisors should make themselves more accessible to subordinates. This will reduce employee frustration and encourage a more cooperative attitude.

Lack of trust

When the element of trust is questioned in a communication situation, the message being transmitted can be affected. It is important for the supervisor to create an atmosphere of openness, while at the same time maintaining confidence, sincerity, and competence when dealing with subordinates.

Either-or thinking

The working world, as with life itself, is filled with many differences between people and differences in how these people go about performing work. The same goal often can be reached by different methods. As in football, where touchdowns can be scored via the run or the pass, it is usually possible at work to accomplish tasks by using different methods. People who take the rigid "either-or" approach unnecessarily restrict their options by ruling out all other possibilities.

Especially with complex problems, talking with several different individuals is more desirable than making a unilateral decision. Of course, talking with several different individuals usually results in a variety of opinions. The supervisor must then make a selection from among options. Such an approach takes more effort but often results in a better decision. Also, by using the communication device of seeking the opinions of others, the health care supervisor begins to develop the reputation of a participative manager if some of those opinions come from subordinates. Participation is considered a highly desirable management characteristic.

Defensiveness

Some people are seldom approachable and some are unapproachable at certain times. This state of not being approachable is defensive in that people place priority in mounting protective devices to shield themselves in their relations with other people. These individuals are fearful that they will be vulnerable to verbal attack, and thus take defensive measures such as being unwilling to consider points of view other than their own. When people show signs of defensiveness, others find difficulty in communicating. In fact, other people often do not even try because experience indicates that the defensive shell cannot be penetrated.

Hostile attitude

Rather than taking a defensive posture to protect themselves, as is the case with defensiveness, some peo-

ple attack others to protect themselves. This is evident when a hostile attitude is displayed. People who exhibit this characteristic are belligerent and show hatred in their aggressiveness. They often are angry and antagonistic. Subordinates and coworkers do not feel comfortable trying to communicate with the person who exhibits a hostile attitude. The problem with this and other barriers is that necessary communication that influences the organization's effectiveness does not occur. People will hesitate to communicate in this environment because battles so often develop.

Know-it-all attitude

A bothersome barrier, even if not as discomfiting as defensiveness and hostility, is the person who gives the impression of knowing everything. Relatively few people are bothered by an individual with acknowledged expertise in a certain subject even if that person is somewhat obnoxious. However, the person who pretends to know everything about every subject that emerges usually is held in low regard. Others are turned off by this behavior and therefore often do not want to even enter the communication network.

Emotional reactions

Most people will react emotionally to stimuli that deeply affect them. In general, such behavior is considered normal and most others understand that infrequent emotional response goes with the human condition. However, the frequency and degree of emotion shown are important considerations. For example, a person who gets upset nearly every time a change is suggested becomes difficult to work with in a complex health organization where change seems to be endemic to the environment. People who allow their emotions to override rational behavior are troublesome individuals to communicate with. Others often shy away from communicating with people who cry or displace anger easily.

Prejudice or bias

Compared with many barriers addressed in this study, prejudice and bias are subtle and sometimes difficult to identify in people who the evaluator does not know well. People are able to mask their true attitudes and feelings. They believe masking is necessary because prejudice and bias are not received positively in this society. Consequently, the passage of a period of time is often necessary before prejudicial behavior can be verified. The implication for organizational communication is that people who are prejudiced or biased against women and racial minorities, for example, often distort messages transmitted to members of these groups.

Lack of credibility

Often people who show prejudice or bias lose credibility with individuals they work with. Likewise, people exhibiting other personality inadequacies that lead to communication barriers suffer credibility loss because others do not believe that they will be treated fairly by such people.

Particularly among managers and supervisors, personal credibility is a tremendous asset. In practice, having credibility usually means that the supervisor is believable. The credible supervisor can be trusted to look out for individual and collective employee interests.

The subject of credibility does not appear in the management literature as frequently as deserved. The reason for its great importance is that credibility serves as a benchmark for the behavioral and interpersonal relations aspect of the manager's position. So much of the manager's work with other people emerges from the basic cornerstones that form the manager's personality.

Fear of distortion or omission of information

Usually, when credibility is present, the fear of distortion or omission of information is absent. Good interpersonal relations often mean that trust is established at a high level. In this kind of environment people feel good about one another and are not constantly on guard out of fear that they will not be treated fairly. However, when the level of trust is low, people are especially vigilant to ensure that others will not take advantage of them.

Lack of interest in the subject matter

Lack of interest in the subject matter is a difficult barrier to overcome. How does one person help another become interested? After informing about the subject, stating its place in the immediate environment, and pointing out the consequences if a task is not accomplished, there is little that another person can do. Often lack of interest is a reflection of poor motivation or a poor attitude.

People must essentially motivate themselves. Sometimes lack of interest is translated accurately as lack of caring. Very important, for example, is the need for the supervisor hiring a new employee to identify whether the prospective employee cares about doing a good job. This matter is so critical in our modern organizations that John Gardner, former Secretary of the U.S. Department of Health, Education and Welfare and founder of the citizen lobby, Common Cause, describes it as one of nine ways to prevent organizational decay.[1]

Personality conflicts

People working in organizations should not be concerned that person-

---

People working in organizations should not be concerned that personality conflicts exist. Alarm need only be registered when these conflicts are disruptive to the organization.

---

ality conflicts exist. Alarm need only be registered when these conflicts are disruptive to the organization. With all the diversity among people and their backgrounds in the modern health care organization, the astonishment may be that more personality conflicts do not exist. Regardless, as with all matters at work, attention needs to be focused on the impact of human interaction as it influences effectiveness and productivity. After all, people are brought together to work and not necessarily to befriend and love each other. If work evaluation indicators verify a high level of performance, personality conflicts can be tolerated. If not, changes must be made.

Differences in perception

Often, personality conflicts are caused by differences in perception. Personality conflicts are not the only barriers that arise from the interaction of incompatible people. Unlike most other societies, the United States is polyglot. So many different subcultures are integrated into the country's overall fabric that there is little cause to wonder when differences in perception are identified. It is important to realize that differences in perception are not necessarily bad. Even people with the same cultural heritage view phenomena differently. Concern arises when perceptual differences cause problems in the organization. Such difficulties can be overcome through education, communication, and the development of flexibility as a behavioral characteristic.

Prematurely jumping to conclusions

Prematurely jumping to answer a question or to address an issue is often the result of a lack of discipline. Yes, health care supervisors must practice discipline just as other mature adults. Sometimes the casual observer may think that only children need discipline. Children obviously do, but so do adults, even wealthy professional athletes, for example. When a hockey referee has already called a penalty against an opponent, the disciplined player does not retaliate. Certainly, on occasion, even the disciplined hockey player fights back in an emotional outburst. Also, as a human being, the health care supervisor is allowed an infrequent aberration.

Specifically regarding the point of prematurely jumping to conclusions, the supervisor must wait until the other person has finished talking or wait until facts or information can be checked. This is the kind of situation in which it is best to count to ten before responding. It is important to know that supervisors do not always have to respond instantaneously. However, they do have to respond in a timely manner.

The difference lies in the nature of the problem. If the supervisor observes an employee abusing equipment, the response has to be immediate. If the problem has to do with the number of hours worked by an employee seeking to qualify for a bene-

fit, the personnel department may have to be contacted and records reviewed. Often this type of problem takes a few days to resolve.

Physical noise and distractions

The job of the supervisor is difficult enough without having to communicate with workers in the midst of noise and distractions. At least in the health care environment, unlike the environment of some elements of heavy industry, supervisors are usually able to ask employees to step to an area free of noise and distractions to talk. This lets the supervisor secure the attention of the worker and be assured that the message is understood. Trying to shout above noise is acceptable only in an emergency.

A far greater danger in the health environment on a day-to-day basis is the chance of the supervisor speaking to employees in locations where patients and other employees can hear. It is absolutely essential that supervisors not reprimand employees in front of patients and other employees unless the offending behavior is causing immediate danger. It is often positive to praise in front of other people but never to condemn except under extenuating circumstances. Human beings lose face when their errors are exposed to other people who have no need to know. Resentment and hostility toward the unthinking supervisor often results.

Overload of too much information

Health care supervisors, like other people who deal with an audience, must understand the audience. Understanding the audience is the best help in determining the amount of information to convey. It may be true that the lower the position in the organizational hierarchy, the less information a person needs to complete a job. This would certainly seem to be true about general organizational information. Within this context, then, workers do not need as much information as managers. The difficulty lies in knowing what information and how much of it to disseminate.

The answer cannot be concrete because each situation is different. Taking time to learn about worker needs and interests is a wise practice to follow. Judgment by the supervisor about the optimum amount of information to communicate is the key. However, judgment cannot be taught in the generic sense. It is always tempered by local factors. The optimum amount of information to convey is known universally to lie only between too much and too little. The point here is not to present too much because it may become dysfunctional and create a barrier for information that is needed. An additional help is to increase the amount of information sent upward to department heads and administrators; they often need to know more about the feelings of employees toward the organization.

Poor organization of ideas

Sometimes employees perceive that too much information is being passed because the items to be communicated are not organized prop-

erly. The solution for this problem is to plan what is to be transmitted after determining what the audience needs and wants and the supervisor decides what actually is to be communicated. The planning process calls for the health care supervisor to think in advance about what to say. For the purpose of organizing ideas, health care supervisors should place themselves in the role of employees for planning purposes, asking, for example, "If I were an employee, what information would be useful and meaningful to me?"

Poor timing of the message

As is true with poorly organized messages, health care supervisors must be sensitive to workers when considering the timing of messages. Simply put, employees can receive messages more effectively at certain times than at others. For example, people probably cannot comprehend additional information as readily when they are under stress to complete a particular job as when they are free of heavy stress. This means that the supervisor should select the most appropriate time to convey messages. Furthermore, supervisors may want to disseminate some information orally and other information in writing. Perhaps appointments, for example, should be written out and given to workers.

Lack of understanding of technical language

Each field and profession seems to develop its own technical language.

Frequently people outside of a particular field or profession have difficulty understanding this technical language. For example, professionals in the health field often talk about HMO (health maintenance organization), PPS (prospective payment system), and PPO (preferred provider organization) as though everybody using the English language knows what is being communicated. This certainly is not the case. The problem is even more acute at lower levels in the organization where workers do not have the need to know much about the emerging concepts in the field. Furthermore, they may not have had formal education in which technical language was studied and discussed.

The solution to the problem has two dimensions that involve audience analysis. One is not to use technical language unless the sender *knows* that the receiver understands. Technical language can often be translated into simple language, and the latter should be used when understanding is known to be limited. The other part of the solution is to educate people to understand the technical language. Although educational programs can be costly and time consuming, supervisors may find that devoting resources for such a purpose is necessary to achieve objectives.

Informal social groups or cliques

People are going to form informal social groups on the basis of mutual interests and compatible personali-

ties. It is only when these groups become counterproductive and degenerate into cliques that supervisors need to become concerned. While thinking supervisors want their employees to get along with each other and develop respect for one another, they do not want groups of employees conflicting with each other and developing rivalries. Sometimes the distinction between acceptable and unacceptable behavior is unclear.

Sometimes the distinction between acceptable and unacceptable behavior is unclear.

The only meaningful practical solution is for health care supervisors to monitor their employees and to frequently gauge the overall level of compatibility.

When supervisors detect that a clique is emerging, it may be well for work assignments to be shifted to break it up. This is another instance in which judgment must be used. No textbook answer applies. However, the supervisor may want to discuss the issue and implications with a progressive personnel manager or supportive manager.

Use of profanity

Due to the nature of the health care field, perhaps problems with the use of profanity are not as severe as in some other industries. However, profanity is offensive to some people. Not only staff members but patients as well may be bothered. If they are bothered, then the use of profanity becomes counterproductive to work, in the case of staff, and to healing, in the case of patients. While a case could possibly be made for the occasional use of profanity to draw attention or to serve as a tool to display emotional interest, overall there seem to be too many negatives for profanity to be considered at all legitimate.

Physical distance between sender and receiver of information

The actual distance between the sender and receiver of information can create problems in communication. This distance factor affects two-way communications, particularly when it involves the supervisor–subordinate relationship. Often subordinates feel alienated from the normal flow of communications. Supervisors need to remember to develop a climate that encourages the flow of information. They need to recognize the value of giving proper feedback to messages in a timely manner no matter how far the distance may be.

Overly competitive attitude

In any organization that generates income, competition usually adds to the productivity and successfulness of the organization. However, when employees within the organization compete too much with each other, then problems can result. Supervisors need to be aware of how important a cooperative attitude can be for the organization. They need to en-

courage and reward an open and cooperative work situation. With this type of situation, employees will work together to exchange information with each other in a positive and helpful manner.

Status or position differences

In any organization, each employee has a role to fill. Whether the employee is a supervisor or subordinate, the role each plays affects the behavior of that individual. This behavior affects communication style. For example, a subordinate may not send information upward because it might be perceived negatively by the supervisor. Supervisors must recognize that this behavior is inherent in the supervisor–subordinate relationship. They need to create an atmosphere of openness and honesty with their subordinates. Such an atmosphere encourages respect for employee views and increases the probability of productivity and job satisfaction.

Poor spatial arrangements

Improper use of space in an organization can contribute to communication problems. The furniture, partitions, equipment, and overcrowding and immobility in the office can restrict eye contact, prevent effective feedback, and generally promote an uncomfortable work environment. When these environmental situations cause communication problems, effective communicators need to remedy the situation by removing the physical barriers, if possible. Consider the needs of employees before making the change, and encourage their input in the planning of the change. Increased participation and improved communication will be the result.

Inability to understand nonverbal communication

When one person speaks to another face to face, more than words are communicated. Frequently, unspoken words or actions are sent along with the spoken message. This unspoken aspect is nonverbal communication. Often what one may say may be contradicted by the actions of the individual. When words and actions are in conflict, communication problems arise. Effective communicators need to be mindful of the nonverbal cues being sent consciously or unconsciously by the receiver of a message. Whether the nonverbal cues are facial expressions, posture, body movements, gestures, and so on, one needs to be aware of these cues so that the message is interpreted and understood the way it was intended.

Speaking too loudly

Few things are more distracting than hearing two people speaking loudly in a heated discussion. Usually when one person increases vocal volume, the other responds with even more volume. When this situation occurs, listening is affected. Individuals concentrate on making their own point without giving consideration to the other's point of view. Increased volume will never get the message across more effectively. When this situation arises, the discussion should be delayed until both parties can deliver their messages in a normal conversational tone.

Lack of health care knowledge

No two people are the same. Each possesses a unique personality based on a different background, set of experiences, education, and so on. Therefore, each individual brings different knowledge to each situation, and this difference will have an effect on message interpretation. Supervisors must not make the mistake of assuming that subordinates with whom the supervisors are communicating possess the same degree of understanding regarding a particular health care concept. This problem occurs frequently when supervisors are involved in training. Often they forget that the subordinates do not have as clear an understanding of the material, therefore causing the subordinates to become anxious and frustrated. The effective supervisor will explain messages fully by giving the appropriate background and supplying additional information necessary to enable the subordinate to understand the message clearly.

Inappropriate physical appearance

The physical appearance of a sender often affects communication because of the impression that appearance makes on the receiver. All the physical aspects of dress, hygiene, hair style, and so on can affect the way one receives a message. What happens is that the receiver may concentrate on the appearance and not listen attentively, be disinterested, or even avoid contact entirely. The effective communicator must always be neat and clean and dress appropriately for the situation.

Training in communications

In the study respondents were also asked how valuable it would be to have additional training in communications. Ninety-one percent of respondents wanted additional training in written communications. However, 99 percent of the participants wanted additional training in both oral and interpersonal communications. Obviously these results suggest the importance of additional communications training in the health care industry.

•   •   •

The results of this study indicate that several barriers to effective communication exist in the health care supervisor–subordinate relationship. These results indicate the particular barriers that should be analyzed and evaluated further by the health care industry. This may be extremely important, especially for those involved in health care training. These barriers, as they relate to the supervisor–subordinate relationship, could be used as a basis for seminars, workshops, noncredit courses, or perhaps presentations at local, regional, or national health care meetings.

Furthermore, seminars for health care personnel should identify models that can be used to maintain and improve relationships between supervisors and subordinates. Topics such as creating a supportive and open environment, along with proper supervisory management coaching techniques, could help to improve the organizational climate for all concerned.

REFERENCE

1. Gardner, J. "How to Prevent Organizational Dry Rot." Presentation to University of Wisconsin Nursing Students, Madison, Wisconsin, 1966.

Making upward communication work for your employees: channels, barriers, and the open door (part 1 of 3)

Charles R. McConnell
Vice President for Employee Affairs
The Genesee Hospital
Rochester, New York

AIRING HER frustrations to a friend and colleague, a registered nurse states, "I'm tired of trying to get answers from nursing administration. Whenever I ask a question that means anything—usually something important to me—I don't seem to get an answer. Usually the first, last, and only thing I hear is, 'We'll get back to you.' All I've learned is that there's no point in asking at all."

Consider also the attitude and outlook of the accountant who has reason to say, "It shouldn't take a week to ten days for me to get to see my boss for a few minutes. He comes and goes a dozen times a day, and when he's here he makes it plain that he doesn't like to be interrupted. Yet at every staff meeting we can count on him to say, 'Don't forget, my door is always open.' Who is he kidding?"

Chances are that in both organizations where the foregoing comments might have been delivered most of

Health Care Superv, 1986,4(4),75–85
© 1986 Aspen Publishers, Inc.

the top managers believe that communication with workers is fairly good, and most middle- and lower-level managers believe that they communicate well with their direct-reporting employees. Hardly a manager at any organizational level will voluntarily concede to being anything less than average or better than average at communication. Perhaps most persons believe themselves better at communication than they really are.

That which employees think and feel—information largely known only to the extent that it is willingly communicated upward by employees—always raises a few unanswerable questions. Although top management will usually concede the presence of more complaints, problems, and unmet needs in the work force than meet the eye or ear, it is not unusual for top management to consistently underestimate the extent of communications problems in the ranks simply because no calamitous events are occurring.

The intent of this discussion is to examine the primary means by which employees communicate with their supervisors and higher management. Much of what follows focuses on those lines and channels of organizational communication that operate least effectively.

The lines and channels of communication within an organization constitute a complex network of thoroughly interrelated paths and processes that include *informal* as well as *formal* channels, *unstructured* as

well as *structured* communication processes, and directions of flow from pure *downward* to pure *upward*.

FORMAL AND INFORMAL CHANNELS OF COMMUNICATION

A work organization of even moderate size includes many formal and informal channels of communication; the number of these channels far exceeds the number of employees in the organization. Strictly formal channels are clearly defined by established organizational relationships; these mostly involve authority relationships between the persons at each end of each channel. For example, the registered nurse reports to the head nurse, the head nurse reports to the day nursing supervisor, the day nursing supervisor reports to the associate director of nursing, the associate director of nursing reports to the vice president for nursing, and the vice president for nursing reports to the president of the institution. This description could, of course, be extended to mention that the president reports to the board of directors.

Between each of the pairs of individuals in the nursing chain of command is an authority relationship that defines the path along which certain information flows. In most of the pairings more channels exist in one direction than in the other. The registered nurse has but one primary, formal, upward channel, that leading to the head nurse. The head nurse, however, may have 20, 30, or more formal downward channels, each defining a formal communicating relationship with one staff nurse in the unit. Thus every person in the organization has a single primary upward channel (except in the case of the rare and frequently troublesome split-reporting relationship in which one person reports to two higher managers), and almost every person who works in a managerial capacity has multiple downward channels, equal to the number of direct-reporting employees.

Within the organization there are also a large number of lateral or roughly lateral channels that might be conveniently referred to as semiformal channels. These channels do not operate in response to direct authority relationships but on a basis of cooperation. This cooperation is implicitly or explicitly mandated but is cooperation nevertheless. Consider, for example, the relationship that might exist in an institution between the payroll department, which is a part of the finance division, and the human resources department, which reports to the operations division, on the seemingly simple matter of processing employment and income verifications for employees who have applied for mortgage loans. Such requests ordinarily enter the organization in the human resources department, which must verify each affected employee's position, title, work status (full time or part time), and duration of employment. Human resources must then request payroll information concerning the employ-

ee's earnings. No direct-reporting relationship exists between payroll and human resources; however, each department is expected by the organization to supply the kinds of information requested by the other and to do so in a reasonable time and manner. When one considers all the departments in an organization that are unrelated to each other in terms of authority relationships but that nevertheless do business with each other regularly, it becomes easy to appreciate the large number of semiformal channels that exist.

While formal and semiformal channels exist by virtue of authority relationships and organizational expectations, informal channels exist through social relationships. An individual's informal channels of communication are as many as the speaking contacts he or she has within the organization. Passing the time of day in social conversation, dealing in rumors, gossip, and other small talk, and griping about one thing or another to anyone who will listen are examples of informal channels of communication. The network of all informal channels is, of course, that well-known carrier of information and misinformation commonly referred to as the grapevine.

The lines separating the various communication channels are not always clear-cut. For example, the supervisor who engages in a bit of talk about the weather with an employee before making an assignment or asking a job-related question is communicating through both formal and informal channels. Likewise, the secretary who today places an order for typewriter service through a purchasing assistant and tomorrow calls that same person to pass along a bit of gossip is operating on both semiformal and informal channels. Thus formal and informal channels are defined not only by authority relationships or lack thereof but also by whether the information carried is work related.

The formal channels of primary concern in this discussion are those that carry information upward, especially those leading from rank-and-file employees to their first-line supervisors.

FORMAL CHANNELS: STRUCTURED AND UNSTRUCTURED

Structured channels have formal mechanisms calling for employee and management participation in specific processes intended to achieve certain results. A primary example of a structured formal channel of upward communication is an organization's *grievance procedure.* Whether in a union or nonunion environment, a grievance procedure exists so that employees can seek redress for perceived improper treatment, endeavor to have certain complaints heard by management, or perhaps challenge certain decisions of management. The procedure is structured in the sense that usually printed forms must be used, specific steps must be taken, and a prescribed timetable must be observed. Pro-

cesses such as the grievance procedure are ordinarily implemented only after attempted resolution by less-structured means has been unsuccessful.

An *employee suggestion program,* in which employee ideas for improving productivity and instituting other changes are transmitted upward, is also a structured formal channel, as are *performance appraisal programs* and *employee surveys. Quality circles* and *work simplification teams* may also be described as structured formal channels because they operate in a more or less prescribed manner to transmit employee thoughts and contributions up the chain of command.

The formal channels that operate upward without benefit of printed forms or prescribed procedures are the unstructured channels. These unstructured channels exist in abundance in the ongoing relationship between employees and their supervisors and all others with whom they are in contact on the institution's business; unstructured channels exist as well in the open-door policy that is frequently espoused by higher management. Information may flow from employee to supervisor by memo, by status report or progress report, or simply by oral feedback; may be shared by the employee who has a need to communicate some information to the supervisor; or may be required as feedback resulting from the supervisor's delegation of tasks to the employee. An unstructured formal channel is also activated whenever an employee takes advantage of a stated open-door policy to carry questions or concerns to higher management.

Communication within a work organization moves downward with far greater ease than it moves upward.

DOWN EASILY, UP WITH DIFFICULTY

Communication within a work organization moves downward with far greater ease than it moves upward. The downward channels of communication are largely controlled by management and are exercised at management's option. Letters and memoranda to employees, employee meetings and staff meetings, informational notes in paycheck envelopes, bulletin boards (except occasional boards devoted solely to employee use), policy and procedure manuals, most newsletters and employee newspapers, and public address systems all represent downward channels of communication controlled by management. Perhaps the most potent downward channels reside in the organizationally vested authority that each level of management has over its subordinates.

When a bit of information is set in motion in any of the downward channels, it moves (barring occasional breakdowns in information flow) as does anything that moves from higher to lower—as though readily assisted by gravity. However, upward communication—moving a message up the chain of command—is often like attempting to make a physical object rise in defiance of gravity.

To obtain communication from employees, the supervisor can and indeed should, through proper delegation, build in requirements for all reasonable forms of employee feedback. That is, if an employee clearly understands that he or she is to report to the supervisor on a given matter at a given time, then reporting usually takes place. In all probability a large part of the effective first-line supervisor's time is consumed in the basic management function of *controlling*—ensuring, through regular follow-up and correction, that work is getting done as intended. This function requires employee feedback.

However, a considerable amount of information can never be secured by the supervisor by mandating feedback through proper delegation. Information that frequently remains hidden from the supervisor includes employee problems (perhaps personal but often also work related) problems experienced with management and coworkers, difficulties in understanding or adhering to certain policies and practices, ideas for improvement that employees may not know how to structure or transmit, complaints about treatment from the organization, and numerous other indications of unmet needs. These kinds of information may be helpful, if not necessary, to the supervisor in running the department, yet the supervisor may obtain such information not through mandate but only by earning the trust and confidence of the employees to the extent that they will volunteer such information.

The barriers that hinder upward communication—in effect, the components of the figurative gravity that impedes the rise of information in an organization—include the following:

- *Physical and organizational distance.* If, for example, the employee and the supervisor are located on different floors or in different structures or if they are assigned to separate facilities with one being housed in a distant satellite, both have built-in communication problems. Much of what should go upward does not go upward because of the difficulty of reaching the supervisor, a situation further complicated if the supervisor is not readily available by telephone. A message that must travel a long organizational distance—a number of steps both laterally and vertically through a complex organizational structure—frequently will not be communicated at all.
- *The number of levels information must travel.* Organization size and complexity provide further barriers to the upward flow of information when many levels in the hierarchy must be traversed. The more levels a message must rise through, the higher the probability of distortion and delay.

- *The attitude of the supervisor.* Regardless of statements such as, "If you have a problem, just look me up," it is the supervisor's day-to-day attitude that determines whether employees do in fact seek out the supervisor. A genuinely open, nonthreatening attitude, of course, inspires trust and confidence and results in vital employee communication. Just as surely, however, a protective or defensive attitude erects barriers that impede upward communication.
- *The supervisor's resistance to involvement.* If a supervisor projects unwillingness to take on more problems or problems that might seem to belong to others, or if he or she seems impatient when listening to what at first might seem to be mostly a personal problem, further barriers to upward communication are erected. Not often will an employee return to a clearly unsympathetic listener.
- *The supervisor's perceived shortage of time.* Most supervisors are unusually busy people, and some often lose sight of the vital need to nurture the face-to-face relationship with each employee. Meetings to attend, projects to work on, letters and memos to write, important reading to wade through—the weight of these and other demands is frequently reflected in perceived time pressure that leads to shorting the employees of the supervisor's

time. The employee who has come to see the supervisor on a matter of some importance will likely not return under similar circumstances if he or she is shuffled out after a five-minute audience during which the supervisor looks at the clock three or four times.

- *No action forthcoming on previous information.* This must stand as one of the most formidable barriers to upward communication. Employees who send their questions and concerns up the chain of command only to get nothing in response sooner or later stop trying to communicate upward. A single item that is swallowed up in the system and never responded to can be more damaging to an organization than a dozen questions for which employees receive answers with which they are unhappy. This barrier is erected over time as management fails to respond to employees' questions. Eventually, the questions stop, and some managers are lulled into believing things are fine in the ranks because nobody is complaining or asking questions. This barrier is overcome only by spending a great deal of time and effort ensuring that all employee communications are answered. Even when no acceptable response can be offered—which is often the case—the supervisor can at least state that no answer is possible and explain why this is

so. This response at least closes the loop in the communications process and lets the employee know that he or she has not been ignored. (Of course, if every response to an employee is of the kind just described, then management has another problem.)

Not all problems related to upward communication can be blamed on the supervisor and the organization; a number of barriers to upward communication originate with employees and must be considered. These include

- *Perceived lack of freedom to call on the supervisor.* The communication that takes place within the context of the supervisor–employee relationship can hardly be described as an equal two-way exchange. The supervisor, as the boss, is permitted by the authority relationship of supervisor over employee to call upon the employee at will and consume the employee's time. However, the employee is far more likely to feel that he or she lacks the freedom to approach the supervisor and command some of the supervisor's time.
- *An authority gap.* When bringing a question, problem, or complaint to the supervisor, the employee is in a position of having to sell something to a person of greater authority. While the supervisor need simply make a statement to the employee and expect acceptance, the employee

faces the uphill struggle of convincing the supervisor.

- *Lack of communications facilities.* The supervisor can use most of the means of downward organizational communication mentioned earlier; but the employees must rely on simple means—oral presentation, pen and paper, and in some cases, for those who have access, typewriter.
- *Possible language barriers.* Although the entire work force is steadily becoming more educated, the individual employee who has a message to convey will probably not be as articulate as the persons for whom the message is intended.
- *Fear of negative consequences.* Some employees will avoid bringing complaints to the supervisor or will soften bad news or bury it altogether rather than risk the supervisor's displeasure.
- *Influence of feelings on facts.* Some employees attempt to communicate with management primarily when they are angered or aggrieved. When negative emotions arise—for example, when a perhaps otherwise legitimate complaint is aired angrily and aggressively—emotion frequently overrides fact, and a number of emotional barriers to communication are erected.
- *Bias against authority.* Regardless of how much an organization may do to ensure open and active lines of communication, a minority of individuals will always

hold back their questions and concerns from management because of a bias against authority. This bias takes two principal forms. In one form, in spite of anything that management as a body and the supervisor as an individual can do, the employee, acutely aware that the boss is always an authority figure, remains shy about initiating contact. Like the timid child intimidated by the adult or the new army recruit who is automatically intimidated by the stripes of the sergeant or the bars of the lieutenant, some persons (thankfully a relative few) do not grow beyond being automatically intimidated by the boss (whoever that may be). The other form of bias against authority (also projected by a relative few in the work force) is distrust of authority of all kinds. To an employee who thinks this way, the authority figure is not to be trusted, workers do the work and "bosses don't do anything," and concerns are not to be carried to the supervisor.

THE OPEN DOOR AND THE CHAIN OF COMMAND

Now and again one hears the claim that the frequently espoused open-door policy is inconsistent with the necessary observance of an organization's chain of command. After all, such reasoning goes, if the individual feels free to go straight to the top of the organization or to any intervening level and be heard, the authority of the immediate supervisor and others in that chain of command is undercut.

Those entering organizational life learn early about the chain of command and the necessity of adhering to that well-marked path. Small wonder that any number of supervisors and managers believe that an open-door policy does no more than circumvent the chain of command. However, the chain of command and an open-door policy are not incompatible if management properly uses the information that arrives by way of the open door. The open-door policy goes awry when higher management, hearing a complaint from a rank-and-file employee, unilaterally alters a decision or conducts an investigation without the knowledge and participation of the intervening managers in the chain of command.

In many organizations that espouse an open-door policy, and in others that have an open-door policy without calling it such, many employees feel free to take their problems and complaints straight to the top. Some will, at their first twinge of discontent, go directly to the top without touching base at lower levels; others will go to the top only after attempting resolution and meeting frustration at lower management levels. Upper management should handle such information by sending the issues—and the persons who brought those issues to the top—to the appropriate points in the chain of command in an attempt at effecting resolution.

The chief executive officer who re-ceives an open-door visit should devote the necessary time to listening to the employee. In the process of conversation with the employee, the chief executive officer should determine whether the employee has told the immediate supervisor of the problem or whether the supervisor is at least aware of the difficulty. If not, the chief executive officer should ask the employee to approach the supervisor directly. The top manager should then pass down the line the information that the employee's immediate supervisor, the supervisor's superior, and possibly the appropriate person in the human resources department will be hearing from the employee on this particular matter. The chief executive officer should make it plain that he or she is not taking sides in the dispute, is neither endorsing nor rejecting the employee's claim, and is not presuming to step in and usurp any functions of other members of management. The chief executive officer is only ensuring that the employee receives the fair and equal treatment available to all employees under organization policies.

If the organization has a grievance procedure, and if the chief executive officer is designated as the ultimate step in the grievance process, he or she should clearly state to the employee at the outset that the executive cannot become intimately involved in the details of the employee's complaint because to do so could compromise the top manager's position should a formal grievance arise later. The top manager will simply guide the employee toward the proper steps for the resolution of all such matters. Above all, the chief executive officer should keep a completely open mind, realizing that he or she is hearing only one side of the issue—and possibly an emotionally colored side at that.

Certainly an effective open-door policy can seem to place a certain amount of pressure on the supervisor and create some risk. However, the

---

An effective open-door policy can seem to place a certain amount of pressure on the supervisor and create some risk.

---

supervisor should understand that it is quite possible—and, indeed, only human—to miss some problems in the work group or, under the pressure of deadlines or the crush of business, to fail to appreciate the full extent of the importance of an issue to a particular employee. In addition, the chief executive officer should understand the supervisor's position and should realize that, for whatever reasons, the employee may have completely bypassed the supervisor and all others.

Admittedly much of the effective operation of an open-door policy lies in the hands of the high-level managers. If the high-level manager enters the process with a truly open mind and is clearly impartial in the face of the difficulty, then the process can be rendered minimally threatening to the supervisor. However, there

is always the likelihood that the supervisor will feel threatened if the supervisor knows he or she can be bypassed by an employee at any time.

If an organization's open-door policy is working correctly,

- every employee will know that he or she can and will receive a fair hearing;
- every supervisor will know that employee information received directly by higher management will not automatically be used contradictorily or punitively but will be pursued with honest concern; and
- ultimately, no one will circumvent the chain of command—the employee will go directly to the immediate supervisor even if the issue or complaint lies with other elements of the organization, and the supervisor will help in effecting resolution.

As suggested earlier, hardly a manager exists who has not at one time or another said, "My door is always open." However, supervisors and managers can project attitudes indicating that, for all practical purposes, the door is closed, including

- displaying obvious annoyance when an employee brings forth a matter of concern;
- criticizing the employee for bringing the matter forth or judgmentally assessing the employee's state of mind ("Calm down—you shouldn't feel that way.");
- displaying obvious impatience with the employee's concern,

creating the impression that the supervisor has far more important things to do;

- being frequently unavailable, creating frustration among employees and suggesting they must necessarily go elsewhere in the chain of command to be heard; or
- failing to respond to previously expressed concerns.

Although organizational statements proclaim the existence of the open door and supervisors and managers espouse the open-door policy, the true open door is established through the attitudes and actions of the occupants of the chain of command. The true open door is ultimately defined by employee perceptions and never by words alone.

(Part 2 will explore grievance processes as a formal means of upward communication for individual employees and will consider the advantages and disadvantages of employee surveys as a means of securing upward communication from large numbers of employees.)

Making upward communication work for your employees: the one and the many: grievance procedures and employee surveys (part 2 of 3*)

Charles R. McConnell
Vice President for Employee Affairs
The Genesee Hospital
Rochester, New York

DOES ANY work organization need both a functioning open-door policy and a structured grievance process? Some people would suggest that these communication approaches are at least partly if not largely duplicative and that if one is in place and functioning properly, the other is not required. Some would also suggest that, in the case of a unionized work force, the employee group has surrendered its right to an open-door policy by trading it off for a detailed grievance procedure. However, although the open-door policy and the grievance process may be at least partly duplicative, there is good reason for encouraging and nurturing the presence and functioning of both.

Part 3 will deal with other means available to the supervisor in attempting to stimulate upward communication—"grapevines" and informal leaders, staff meetings, performance appraisal conferences, and individual employee contact.

Health Care Superv, 1986,5(1),81–91
© 1986 Aspen Publishers, Inc.

The major reasons for maintaining both practices include the following:

- The very nature of communication suggests that its improvement and refinement is a never-ending process, and that, in an organization of any appreciable size, communication is never 100 percent perfect.
- No single means of employee communication, no matter how structured, thorough, or conscientiously applied, will always catch everything or encourage all information that is of value to management. However, the more means of communication available, the more pertinent information management will catch overall.
- There will always be some employees who will not use one particular process but will be willing to use the other. Therefore, the more such processes that are available, the greater the number of employees who will take advantage of the opportunities for upward communication.
- The processes can be made to complement each other. Operation of a true open-door policy will permit informal resolution of many difficulties that need not become grievances and will highlight those particular issues that do require closer scrutiny; such a policy will encourage issues to follow the path of formal grievance resolution.

OPEN-DOOR POLICY

For better or for worse, an open-door policy always exists, and it is the first process that is often taken advantage of—simply because it is not a particularly structured approach. However, the addition of a formal grievance procedure is by no means an indication of a failed open-door policy. Both processes are needed. In many ways they are similar, but to an undeniable extent they are different channels of employee communication filling different needs. Because of the differences in how they operate, each catches some of what the other misses.

To this point, the term grievance has been applied as a label for the established process provided for the resolution of certain differences. The process takes its name from the act of grieving, or, to put it simply, complaining about something. Because of the considerable integration of grievance procedures in collective-bargaining agreements, many people have come to associate the mention of a grievance procedure with the existence of a collective-bargaining unit.

In some settings, however, perhaps a more appropriate name than grievance procedure would be appeal procedure. An appeal, roughly defined the same way as is an appeal in the legal sense, is the act of objecting to a decision and asking for its alteration or reversal. Therefore, some organizations, primarily those that are nonunion, have a preference for referring to this particular kind of mechanism as an "appeal procedure," if only because "grievance procedure" carries such a strong collective-bargaining connotation.

The attitude of some management groups is to concede to the necessity for a formal resolution process only when it is required by a collective-bargaining agreement. However, to have such a process only when it is contractually required is to deprive nonunion management of a valuable avenue of employee communication. A formal problem resolution mechanism can do considerable good in any organization, so there is surely no point in waiting for a union to come in and mandate a grievance procedure before agreeing to the presence of such a process. An honest, effectively functioning problem resolution mechanism can also go a long way toward helping a nonunion organization retain that desired status.

A MODEL APPEAL POLICY AND PROCEDURE

The policy and procedure described in this section, while closely resembling the processes used in a number of health care organizations, is both a comprehensive generalization of the kinds of steps that might be found in such a process and a specific model that might apply in and of itself.

Among the most commonly appealed decisions are those that result in employee disciplinary actions and those relating to performance evaluations.

Appealable matters

The first matter to be dealt with in this appeal process is the definition of an appealable matter. First, an employee can appeal a decision of management. Among the most commonly appealed decisions are those that result in employee disciplinary actions and those relating to performance evaluations (in other words, employees may protest their evaluations through the appeal process). An employee can also appeal a manager's interpretation or implementation of a policy of the organization. However, organizational policy itself is not appealable. For example, should the organization's policy call for eight paid holidays per year, an employee cannot exercise the right of appeal to ask for more holidays.

The process

The appeal process is available to any nonmanagerial employee who has passed the basic three-month probationary period and has thus become a regular employee. In most organizations that have such appeal processes in place, members of management are not eligible to appeal.

Following the occurrence of an event that might be considered appealable, the employee has 72 hours (three full working days) in which to file an appeal. This time limit can be extended as necessary to account for employee illness or other circumstances that might prevent the prompt filing of an appeal. However, this filing time limit is never extended without reasonable cause, primarily to ensure that only current matters and not "history" are being appealed. An employee cannot, for example, decide three weeks after receiving an evaluation that he or she considers unfavorable that this evaluation will now be appealed.

This appeal process encompasses either four or five steps, depending on the nature of the action being appealed. Those persons who are involved in evaluating the appeal at each step have three days to complete their step. Likewise, the employee has three days to consider the results of each step and to decide either to accept the findings of that step and discontinue the appeal or to continue the appeal. Any of these three-day periods can be extended if, in the judgment of the human relations officer and with the agreement of the employee, it is decided that more time will be required to facilitate the thorough completion of the step. For example, if a given step requires monitoring a particular activity over a period of a week or so, this will be considered necessary cause, and an extension will be granted. If a key individual in the process happens to be

away on vacation, the process will be suspended until the person returns. Lacking good cause to extend, however, each step and each response must be concluded within three working days.

As already mentioned, an individual in the human resources department, such as an employee-relations officer, an employee advocate, or a corporate ombudsperson, administers the appeal procedure as an interpreter, counselor, and general representative of the employee. It is the initial task of this individual, upon receiving an employee's complaint and learning of the desire to appeal, to ensure that the matter has been thoroughly discussed between employee and supervisor without resolution before proceeding to the formal appeal procedure.

The procedure is implemented upon the employee's provision of an appeal statement written by the employee with the guidance of the employee-relations officer as necessary. At a minimum, this appeal statement must convey

- specifically *what* decision, action, or condition is being appealed;
- *why* this particular decision, action, or condition is being appealed;
- specifically what the employee wishes to accomplish by way of the appeal process. This piece of information is essential to the process; it must be known precisely what the employee desires to obtain from the appeal so that

all attempts at resolution may be oriented in appropriate directions. For example, an individual who is appealing a written warning that he or she may believe is overly punitive may perhaps request that the written warning be reduced to an oral reprimand. As another example, an employee who is being discharged for misconduct might specify reinstatement as the objective or perhaps might ask to be given the right to resign for purposes of the employment record; and

- exhibits or other backup documents as necessary.

Steps of the appeal procedure

First, with the assistance of the employee-relations officer, the employee provides the appeal statement. The employee-relations officer notifies all involved managers of the existence of the appeal and submits the appeal to the employee's immediate supervisor. The supervisor is expected to respond in writing within three working days. This response is channeled through the employee-relations officer to the employee, and the employee decides either to accept or to continue the appeal.

Second, should the employee express the desire to continue, the appeal is then sent to the immediate superior of the supervisor who responded in the first step. Once again a response provided within three working days is returned to the employee through the employee-re-

lations officer, and again the employee is faced with the decision to accept the stated position, to recommend resolution, or to continue the appeal.

Should the appeal continue to the third step, the organization's director of human resources provides a response as appropriate. Once again, within the normal limitations of the three-day turnaround, a response is transmitted to the employee, and the employee makes the decision to accept or continue.

Fourth, should the appeal be continued, it is submitted for consideration to an appeal committee composed of three or four members of executive management (none of whom has yet been called on to judge the appeal) chaired by the director of human resources. This appeal committee's decision is final regarding matters of wages, hours, working conditions, and the like. However, if termination is the subject of the appeal, there is an additional step available to the employee.

The fifth and final step available to an employee being terminated (and in some organizations, employees who have been suspended, resulting in the loss of one or more day's pay) is personal review and consideration of the appeal by the chief executive officer (CEO) of the organization. The CEO will review the results of the preceding four steps and will listen to the employee's personally stated case. In attempting to determine whether there are extenuating circumstances that may have been

> *One of the primary functions of the CEO in the appeal, in addition to displaying a willingness to listen to the employee, is to determine whether the process operating on the employee's behalf has indeed been fair, impartial, and thorough.*

missed or misinterpreted at previous levels, and also looking closely for consistency of policy application and employee treatment, the CEO will seldom overturn the results of the previous steps. One of the primary functions of the CEO in the appeal, in addition to displaying a willingness to listen to the employee, is to determine whether the process operating on the employee's behalf has indeed been fair, impartial, and thorough.

External options

An employee who was terminated and who remains terminated after exhausting the appeal process may also be advised by the employee-relations officer of possible avenues of recourse available outside of the organization. However, the human-relations officer is also obligated to provide the employee with a realistic assessment of how this particular complaint might be viewed outside of the organization.

Frequently, employees who have been discharged go to the Equal Employment Opportunity Commission (EEOC), the State Division of Human Rights, or other outside agencies, claiming that discrimination has been committed. The employee who has taken full advantage of the appeal process is in a better position to pursue a complaint with an outside agency if that employee believes that discrimination has been involved. Conversely, the employee who lodges a complaint with an outside agency without having first exhausted all internal avenues of redress is often on less solid ground in pursuing the complaint.

Should the employee involved in a complaint be a member of a collective-bargaining organization, and if that which has been referred to as an appeal procedure is in fact designated as a grievance procedure, the approach will nevertheless be similar to that which has already been described. There may, however, be variations in the number of steps available and in the amount of turnaround time allowed for each step. Depending on what the collective-bargaining agreement may say, the ultimate step in the grievance procedure could call for submission of the grievance to binding arbitration in which both sides have contractually agreed to accept the final determination of an independent third party.

SUPERVISOR'S APPROACH

At times the employee appeal procedure might seem threatening to the supervisor. However, along with all of the other policies and procedures of the organization, the appeal procedure is but one of a number of forces existing in modern organizational life that encourage the supervisor to act thoughtfully, consistently, and responsibly in matters of importance to employees. In approaching any individual appeal the supervisor should

- be prompt, making every reasonable effort to respond to the appeal within the designated time limits (barring justified extensions of time). However, the supervisor's reply should not be rushed; as much of the available time as necessary should be taken to ensure completion of any necessary investigation and to guarantee careful consideration of the facts;
- gather all available information before responding. Although the supervisor may have felt thoroughly justified in rendering the original decision, the fact that the decision is being appealed has placed it in the spotlight and opened it up to scrutiny. The supervisor should not simply reaffirm the original decision without looking deeply enough into the matter to determine whether anything important might have been missed;
- conscientiously seek to resolve the difficulty to remove this particular matter as a barrier to the employee's willing performance;
- appreciate that hindsight is often revealing, providing a perspective from which the passage of time and the revelation of additional information call for a dif-

ferent view of the problem. The supervisor should be able to admit to a mistake if hindsight suggests that one has been made but should also be prepared to support the original decision if this valuable hindsight simply serves to validate the decision;
- be constantly aware of the need for consistency in the treatment of employees. Consistency of employee treatment is a key in the continuing application of the organization's policies. Barring the presence of clear extenuating circumstances, what applies to one employee should apply equally to all employees;
- if unable to concede to the employee and grant the desired outcome of the appeal, fully explain why this cannot be done. This may do nothing to satisfy the employee, but it will nevertheless discharge the supervisor's obligation to provide the employee with the reasons for the action taken; and
- avoid being sensitive to the point of taking the appeal personally. Certainly an employee appeal is a criticism, but it is a criticism of a supervisory action or decision; it is not, except to the extent that an employee may (erroneously) present the complaint, a criticism of the supervisor personally.

EMPLOYEE SURVEYS

The employee survey represents a thoroughly structured formal channel of upward communication. Structure is necessary because questions must be carefully prepared and mechanisms must be established for collecting and processing responses. However, unstructured surveys are possible—for example, calling for a show of hands in response to a simple question asked at an all-employee meeting would constitute a simple unstructured survey.

As a means of employee communication, all-employee surveys are not without their uses. However, surveys often have associated with them tasks and difficulties that are not always taken into account when the decision is made to survey the employees. On occasion, they are highly useful when dealing with referendum-type issues (issues for which it is clearly to management's advantage to know the position of the employee population as a whole).

Employee surveys range from highly structured, all-encompassing, organizationwide "employee attitude" surveys or "employee opinion" surveys, to extremely narrow and targeted surveys that may deal with a single issue and one small group of employees. The hazards of employee surveys exist in a direct relationship to the scope of the survey; the broader the survey ranges, the greater the hazards are. Thus the broad employee-attitude or employee-opinion surveys tend to be the most hazardous in terms of opportunities for possible negative repercussions.

Problems inherent in surveys

That which is commonly referred to as the employee-attitude survey

may encompass dozens of questions—surveys of 100 or more questions are not uncommon—that deal with all aspects of employment, ranging from the image of the institution overall, through all aspects of employee communication and supervisory behavior, and even including the quality and price of the food in the cafeteria and the adequacy of parking facilities. Such surveys must ordinarily be conducted by convening sizable groups of employees in classroom-style meetings for a sufficient length of time to complete the form, or by mailing a questionnaire to all employees and hoping for the largest possible response. There are problems related to both methods of obtaining responses. Persons who feel uneasy trying to come up with answers will often not bother with a mail-in questionnaire, but some of these same people, if trapped into responding in a classroom setting, will consciously or unconsciously allow their resentment to be reflected in their responses.

There is also the problem of wide variations in individual understanding of survey questions. This problem may be only partly solved by the guidance provided in a survey-completion session. Not all employees share the same level of literacy, and even in the better surveys—those presented in simple declarative statements targeted as closely as possible to the least common denominator of the employee group—some statements will be misunderstood by some employees. As many managers who have worked with surveys have discovered, a group's response to a given survey question can be swayed considerably in either direction by the way that question is worded.

One of the greatest problems inherent in the all-employee survey is that of the expectations created by the survey itself. For a survey to be taken seriously, management must convince employees that it is being undertaken for good reasons. The reasons usually involve management's

---

For a survey to be taken seriously, management must convince employees that it is being undertaken for good reasons.

---

desire to know how good a job it is doing running the organization for its customers, clients, patients, and employees. Management usually also claims that it desires to know what the employees' problems are so management can make things better. Even if this is not a stated objective of such a survey (it usually *is*), it is there loud and clear by implication. Thus all-employee surveys raise employees' expectations of management: Employees expect that if widespread problems are uncovered, management will do something about them.

As far as management is concerned, an all-employee survey strongly suggests that management is, in advance, buying into a commitment to act on the survey's results. However, top management personnel frequently have no idea of what will be revealed by the survey, and they may have

done an effective job of believing that no serious problems exist simply because they have heard of none. They could indeed have been hearing nothing because there was nothing unfavorable to hear. However, it is at least likely, if not more likely, that top management would be hearing nothing unfavorable because the organization's upward channels of communication were not working.

The greatest danger presented by an all-employee survey, then, is that it might be implemented unknowingly in the presence of totally clogged upward channels of communication that are then instantly and very nearly violently blown wide open. When this occurs, management has but two choices: to concede to the difficulties and get busy repairing them, which may be nearly impossible for present management because they will be tagged with responsibility for these difficulties; or to do what some management groups who have been so shocked have done and bury the survey results, or at least the negative parts, and add the employees' expectations to the already considerable underlying discontent in the organization.

Outside consultants

Although many organizations attempt to develop their own survey questions and perform the task entirely without outside assistance, probably the most useful all-employee surveys are conducted by outside consultants. The best survey questions are extremely carefully written, have been tested in practice, and generate results that may be statistically validated. Survey consultants are in a better position to supply survey questions that come with fewer built-in problems.

There are also many questions that can be raised relative to the norms to which a survey's results may be compared. For example, it does only a minimal amount of good if a survey has revealed to management that 12.7 percent of employees believe the institution's pension plan is inadequate. This tells management only that, on the average, 12 to 13 employees out of 100 do not believe the pension plan is adequate. With what may this be compared? Some survey consultants supply, along with the results of a survey, an automatic comparison with norms that may be established along the lines of the industry, the region, or the nation. These norms are generated from the results of other organizations' use of the same survey, and after a period of time, these data may be used to produce norms that are statistically significant.

Some organizations that have repeated their attitude surveys at regular intervals over the years have discovered that the best "norms" to compare with are their own previous survey results. If, for example, this year's survey did indeed indicate that 12.7 percent of employees were dissatisfied with the pension plan, but comparison indicated that this figure was down from a high of 18.5 percent and a 10-year average of 14.8 percent,

then management not only knows exactly where it stands today regarding employee opinion of the pension plan, but it also knows the direction in which its responses to previous years' information has been leading.

Certainly it is costly to keep repeating an employee-attitude survey (two- or three-year intervals are common) to build a significant database; however, a number of organizations have corporately concluded that doing just that is cost-effective over the long run. Indeed, it is likely that almost any health care organization could conduct an attitude survey every two to three years for a period of 10 to 20 years overall without spending as much money as management would be forced to spend in combating one determined union organizing campaign.

The individual supervisor will have little to say about who is selected to conduct the organization's employee attitude survey. However, in an organization that practices true participative management, the supervisor may have the opportunity to express some opinions. If this is the case, serious consideration should be given to recommending an outside attitude survey, with questions thoroughly tested and validated, conducted by experienced survey consultants. And the best source of information as to which consultants do an effective job and which outside surveys are best is the time-honored satisfied customer—other organizations that have utilized these services.

Smaller, specifically focused surveys are considerably safer than full-scale attitude or opinion surveys. Often these can be thoroughly and efficiently accomplished internally. However, some common-sense guidelines should always apply: The issues should be as simply stated as possible, should be conveyed in as few simple statements as possible, and should carry the promise of management follow-up. For example, a hospital of more than 2,000 employees was considering the addition of a supplemental life-insurance program in which people could purchase additional coverage for themselves by payroll deduction. The matter had surfaced only because an insurance company that was endorsed by a number of hospital groups went on the selling trail calling on all hospitals to explain the benefits of one particular program that was essentially traditional life insurance. A number of managers felt that there would be sufficient employee desire to implement such a program. However, when the question of whether term-life coverage had been considered instead of or in addition to whole-life insurance, management could only guess at employee preferences. A survey was suggested. Every effort was made to reach all employees with survey forms distributed through their immediate supervisors. The carefully written survey form

included just five or six simple statements all calling for yes or no responses. These statements were designed to tell management whether those employees who would consider purchasing extra life insurance would prefer to have whole-life, term-life, or both programs. The responses indicated only minimal interest in whole-life insurance but a significant interest in supplemental term-life insurance. Therefore, a supplemental term-life insurance program was implemented, completely opposite from the proposed whole-life insurance program, and more than 40 percent of employees entered into voluntary participation, and management received positive feedback on the decision to make such a program available. Had no survey been conducted, the organization might well have gone forward with the creation of a program based on totally erroneous assumptions about the employees.

•   •   •

Employee surveys can be made to perform a vital function in bringing employee information upward in the organization. However, the price of employee survey participation is usually management's advance commitment to share the results of the survey and to act positively on certain of those results.

Making upward communication work for your employees: processes and people, with emphasis on people (part 3 of 3)

Charles R. McConnell
Vice President for Employee Affairs
The Genesee Hospital
Rochester, New York

THE MOST effective way for any member of a work organization to stimulate incoming communication is to make every effort to ensure that outgoing communication is occurring. This certainly applies to the supervisor who wishes to inspire increased upward communication from the work group. In the process of actively supplying the employees with the means by which to communicate upward, the supervisor is actually communicating downward in a way that increases the likelihood of employees communicating upward.

In stimulating upward communication the supervisor must be able to take advantage of all reasonable means available, whether formal and relatively structured, such as performance appraisal conferences, or informal and unstructured, such as tapping into the office grapevine or dealing with the group's informal leaders, or something in between,

Health Care Superv, 1987, 5(2), 71–80

such as scheduled departmental meetings.

In short, effective employee communication will not occur on its own or by virtue of organizational processes that may be in place. It will occur only if the supervisor takes steps to make it happen.

MAKING CONSTRUCTIVE USE OF THE GRAPEVINE

The communications phenomenon known as the "grapevine" may be described as the communications system of the informal organization. The informal organization is that complex network of interrelationships, determined primarily by social relationships, that overlays the formal organization structure. One is also likely to hear the term "the rumor mill" used to describe the grapevine. However, the grapevine is a rumor mill only part of the time; the grapevine can carry information that is accurate and usable, as well as the significant volumes of misinformation associated with its use. The greatest problems presented by the grapevine are embodied in the difficulties of trying to separate truth from untruth and useful from useless and harmful, and in the impossibility of completely controlling the flow of any of these kinds of information.

Were one to post a notice proclaiming the immediate abolition of the grapevine and a total prohibition of further use of this means of communication, one might well be laughed out of the organization. It is clearly not possible to shut off the flow of information that travels through informal relationships. However, the amount of information that flows through the informal organization bears an inverse relationship to the amount of information that flows through the formal organization; that is, as the volume of information flowing through formal channels decreases, the amount of information traveling via informal channels increases.

The individual supervisor—and for that matter, every member of management up to and including the chief executive officer—is a grapevine participant. All of these people, through their social relationships within the organization, are members of the informal organization. Even outside of direct reporting relationships or other working relationships they talk with others about many matters relevant to the organization.

The better the state of employee communications within the organization, the smaller the amount of misinformation carried by the grapevine.

Essentially, all that can be said about fostering effective employee communications can be related to the control of the grapevine. The better the state of employee communications within the organization, the smaller the amount of misinformation carried by the grapevine. Whether the grapevine will flourish in a negative sense in one's own department less than in the overall organization is determined by the overall communications posture of the supervisor. Rarely will one be able to stamp out rumors and misinformation completely, but the supervisor can minimize the flow of misinformation by:

- *Remaining visible and available to the employees*—If the supervisor can be readily reached, can be readily accessed by employees who have questions and concerns, some grapevine activity will be avoided. Employees who are unable to communicate their questions and concerns because they cannot talk with the supervisor (who may be off in meetings or serving on committees, away on trips, working constantly with visitors, or may be seemingly glued to a telephone instead of actively supervising), they are then more likely to pass along their concerns in the form of speculation to be carried by the grapevine. Thus, the grapevine becomes the outlet for employees who experience a communications vacuum.
- *Never failing to provide an employee with an answer*—The employee who does not receive a response to an expressed concern may not experience the same frustrations that are associated with the manager who is neither visible nor available. However, the employee so treated is likely to experience even greater frustration created by the supervi-

sor's chronic nonresponse. The employee who continually sees questions and concerns swallowed up in the system eventually stops trying to communicate upward. Every employee deserves—and should receive—an answer or, at the very least, a nonanswer (a reasonable explanation of why a true response is not possible). As with the supervisor's unavailability, a supervisor's chronic nonresponse creates a vacuum that will be filled, usually inadequately, by the grapevine.

- *Being a stopper of rumors and conjecture*—The supervisor will be party to many grapevine transmissions. Many of these transmissions will come through one's own employees; indeed, the supervisor who has the trust and confidence of the work group will hear much current rumor and speculation from the employees in the group. When in receipt of some piece of information that is clearly speculative, rather than pass it along to others or attempt to correct it with more speculation, the supervisor should ask employees to please not pass the story further before it can be checked. Some employees will of course continue transmitting, perhaps even adding the observation that their supervisor had some doubts about the story, but some will comply and will wait until they receive clarification. In brief, the supervisor who picks up rumors should do everything possible to either verify the information or replace it with the correct information. There is no better way for the supervisor to make use of the grapevine than to give it something clear, simply stated, and accurate to carry.

It is necessary to accept the inevitability of the grapevine. It is there, and it will always be there. However, the individual supervisor will remain one of the primary factors in determining whether grapevine transmissions originating within the work group are largely negative or mostly positive. People will always talk with other people, but whenever the grapevine is allowed to take the place of effective employee communication by default, the results can be damaging.

INVOLVING THE WORK GROUP'S INFORMAL LEADERS

Almost every work group has its informal leaders. These people range from highly visible to barely distinguishable from the rest of the work group, depending upon the relative strength of personalities or other characteristics that differentiate them from the rest of the group. Informal leaders are often outgoing individuals who possess some natural leadership traits. The extent to which one may be an informal leader is determined almost entirely by the degree to which others are accepting of that leadership. That is, informal leadership is conferred completely by the followers.

Natural leaders ordinarily differ from most others in the work group in one or more ways that set them apart and cause others to turn to them at certain times. Depending on the particular characteristics involved, an individual may be a natural leader in almost any setting or in only one particular setting. For example, someone who is highly articulate and who is a naturally sympathetic listener may assume an informal leadership role in almost any work group, but someone whose informal leadership is based on technical expertise may possess informal leadership in a group of largely inexperienced people but may simply be one of the crowd if moved into a group of highly knowledgeable and experienced people.

Knowledge and experience relative to the rest of the work group are indeed a pair of the factors that may determine informal leadership. Likewise, being an articulate conversationalist and a sympathetic listener—that is, being a good, natural communicator—points toward informal leadership. In addition, establishing a tendency toward informal leadership are: the outgoing nature of someone who welcomes constant contact with others; the assertive nature of someone more given to initiative and action than to inaction; humanistic traits that cause one to be genuinely concerned about others; and a natural interest and curiosity about what is occurring beyond the scope of one's own daily duties.

Unfortunately, informal leaders may also be people who are basically insecure and are continually seeking affirmation of their worth by striving to remain at center stage; people who are willing to use their apparent influence over others for their own benefit; people who are deliberately seeking power and influence; and people whose frustrated desires to rise within the organization have turned toward seeking other ways to elevate themselves relative to others. It is, of course, reasonably well known that some workers who have failed repeatedly in their quest for promotion (and quite often failed because their perceived skills may have been inadequate, although their drive for advancement was strong) have become internal organizers for unions that wished to represent the employees. Many such people, although they themselves may not be fully aware of the path they have chosen at the beginning of union organizing, have opted to reach for union career ladders because organizational career ladders have been denied them.

The identification of all possible informal leaders within the rank-and-file employee group is always an early objective of a union that is seeking to organize the institution's employees. Therefore, it is important that the supervisor be keenly aware of the informal leaders, especially those employees who seem always to be at the center of conversation in the lunch group or the coffee break group; the ones who cast themselves

in the role of bringing forth the concerns of others and generally as serving as spokespersons for the group; and the ones who are most often cited as sources in grapevine transmissions. Although some informal leaders are and will always remain distrusting of the supervisor's authority and opposed to management in most matters, the majority of informal leaders exhibit a number of positive characteristics that can perhaps be turned toward good effect. It is among the informal leaders, especially those who are such by virtue of knowledge, experience, and natural communications skills, that the supervisor ordinarily finds the best workers to whom important tasks can be delegated.

It is among the informal leaders that the supervisor ordinarily finds the best workers to whom important tasks can be delegated.

In the continuing task of making upward channels of communication function for the employees, the supervisor must consider the group's informal leaders as especially important points of contact within the group. The supervisor who finds it necessary to make constructive use of the grapevine by launching a piece of information on its way or perhaps by setting a rumor straight would do well to begin with the group's informal leaders. Others, through their contact with the informal leaders and each other, will get the message. Ideally, of course, the supervisor should hold every employee in the group in equal regard and not single out some for favored communication treatment. However, some employees, no matter how well or fairly they are treated, will not come forward and deal with the supervisor directly, but they will usually deal with the informal leaders. Thus, some employees will receive some information through the informal leaders, and they are thus more likely to reciprocate in passing their concerns to the informal leaders. And the informal leaders, unlike those few employees who rarely come forward, will willingly bring matters to the attention of the supervisor. The supervisor who is fair and open with the entire work group and who deals honestly with the group's informal leader will find that the informal leaders are valuable facilitators of upward communication for the entire group.

DEPARTMENTAL STAFF MEETINGS

Departmental staff meetings should be held at regularly scheduled intervals. The frequency of such scheduled meetings can vary according to the type of department involved and how much regularly accumulated information there is to be shared with all employees. Perhaps an active personnel department or accounting department would find that every one or two weeks would not be too often to hold a staff meeting. For certain other departments, however,

for example, a maintenance department or a food service department, a quarterly meeting might be sufficient for getting all of the employees in the group together (although certain smaller segments of the department would certainly meet more frequently). For the larger departments, such as the department of nursing, a quarterly staff meeting might be held by bringing a number of subgroups together at various times over a 24- or 48-hour period so that all department members on all shifts might be covered without either pulling all staff off the units at the same time or creating such a large single group that little true information exchange could be accomplished.

Regardless of the interval, it is important that employees expect to attend staff meetings at a regularly scheduled time. When staff meetings are scheduled on an ad hoc basis and held irregularly, perhaps in the belief that one need schedule a staff meeting only when there is something significant to deal with, they tend not to be held for long periods of time. They tend also to occur, under this mode of scheduling, only for important—and usually bad—news or when major problems have developed. Thus, employees tend to become shy of staff meetings, because they have learned that under these circumstances such meetings mean unpleasant developments.

Not every regularly scheduled staff meeting should have to deal with a full agenda of significantly consequential information. Rather, occasional meetings that are brief and deal with routine, nonstressful items can provide a welcome break for employees while fully serving one of the primary purposes of staff meetings: fostering the communicating relationships between and among supervisor and employees.

A departmental staff meeting should be a two-way exchange of information and ideas. Certainly there will be announcements and items of information to be passed from supervisor to employees, but even these should be subject to questioning and discussion and never couched in the form of one-way statements. (Regarding announcements that the supervisor might consider routine, it is far too easy to give way to the tendency to play television newscaster and simply deliver them in a cut and dried one-way fashion that discourages interchange.)

It is highly preferable for staff meetings to include individual reports and discussion items presented by members of the group. One might report on attendance at a seminar on a topic of interest to the group; others might report on the status of projects or problems in which they are involved. However, such reports must be prearranged with the people who are going to deliver them. This prearrangement is necessary for two reasons. First, the person who will be expected to speak and perhaps to deal with the questions of others should have time for proper preparation. Second, many rank-and-file employees do not have a supervisor's ex-

perience in talking with groups of people and are sometimes shy and fearful about doing so.

To "trap" someone into speaking before the group will often inspire resentment in the person so trapped. A reasonably small group that meets frequently under the direction of a supervisor who is sensitive to the needs of individuals will eventually find itself operating in a friendly, nonthreatening, informal environment in which most people will speak up. However, almost every group has its members who are frightened—almost deathly so—of speaking before a group of people, and these persons must be drawn out slowly and understandingly without being put on the spot. The more open, friendly, and informal the group can be in its operation (and it is certainly possible to be all of these while still observing a reasonable agenda), the more likely it is that everyone, or nearly everyone, will participate.

Many topics are fair game for a departmental staff meeting agenda. However, the supervisor should discourage the airing of individual personality conflicts or disputes involving problems of working relationships within small groups of employees. The supervisor should seek to avoid the airing of difficulties that amounts to employees telling on each other in the group setting. The staff meeting should remain primarily the forum for the discussion of work-related matters that are relevant to the group as a whole.

Properly administered, the departmental staff meeting is a powerful forum for employees' upward communication of information. If the meeting's atmosphere is friendly and nonthreatening, and if meetings are held regularly so that people are accustomed to them, staff are most likely to participate to the fullest extent.

PERFORMANCE APPRAISAL CONFERENCES

One of the primary purposes of a performance appraisal interview is to give the employee the opportunity for immediate feedback on the appraisal. Of course, in most organizations the performance appraisal and a subsequent interview are required. Although this contact may be mandated, the supervisor should never regard the appraisal interview as a requirement to be dispensed with in as little time as possible, but rather should take advantage of this opportunity to hold a wide-ranging conversation concerning the employee's view of his or her performance as well as that performance as reported in the appraisal.

All that might be said about the proper way to hold a performance appraisal conference is applicable to this discussion of upward communication. The performance appraisal is a formal, fairly structured channel of upward employee communication, and it should be used to the fullest possible extent along with all other available means of providing the em-

ployee with opportunities to talk with the supervisor on employment-related matters.

The performance appraisal interview will provide a great deal of information about the state of the communicating relationship between the supervisor and the individual employee. The greater the number of surprises, disappointments, and controversies that arise in an appraisal interview, the shakier is the state of the relationship between the supervisor and that employee. Conversely, the fewer difficulties that arise in an appraisal interview the better the state of the communicating relationship between the two parties. In the ideal situation—that is, when the ongoing communicating relationship between supervisor and employee is all that it should be or can be—the appraisal interview will be no more than a pleasant formality, because the two parties will already know completely where they stand with each other on all matters.

ONE-TO-ONE DISCUSSIONS

Any employee in the group should be able to access the supervisor through the normally open door. This should be permitted on as nearly a random basis as possible, providing the employee uses reasonable discretion in determining when to ask the supervisor for a few minutes of time. Such conversations should be established by appointment only when arranging to bring two equally busy people together on an important matter, or when it is clear that the matter to be discussed could take considerable time. The employee should of course always inquire if the time is right for a brief discussion and offer to do so by appointment if the moment of asking is inappropriate for some legitimate reason.

As a matter of maintaining continuing availability, supervisors should make it a habit to intermittently engage employees in individual conversation when opportunities to do so present themselves.

Some employees, however, will rarely if ever exercise the open door, and some will never approach the supervisor even at times when they clearly should be doing so. As a matter of maintaining continuing availability, supervisors should make it a habit to intermittently engage employees in individual conversation when opportunities to do so present themselves. For example, if an employee stops at the supervisor's door to drop off an awaited document or orally deliver a brief message, the supervisor might say, "If you have a few minutes to spare, have a seat and let's talk about how things are going in general." Perhaps the encounter brings forth nothing more than a brief exchange of small talk and pleasantries; however, the supervisor has given the employee the opportunity for contact, and providing this oppor-

tunity alone sends a clear message to the employee, in effect: "This supervisor knows I'm around and cares about me and how I'm doing." But it is also fully as likely that the employee will reveal a problem or speak about a complaint or perhaps ask a question that he or she believes to be important.

The supervisor should always be prepared to take advantage of such opportunities to talk with the employees. In addition, the supervisor should also go out of the way to create such opportunities. One might consider simply dropping in at the work station of an employee—preferably at a time when the person is not overburdened—and initiating a friendly conversation that gives the employee the same opportunity to talk with the supervisor informally as a visit to the supervisor's office would have provided. Such behavior on the part of the supervisor, while on rare occasion creating uneasiness on the part of the very few employees who remain forever distrustful of authority and would just as soon be left alone, goes a long way toward promoting the supervisor's visibility and availability and offers employees increased opportunity for upward communication. This approach has occasionally been described as "management by wandering around," and most of the time it serves its purpose well.

To effectively manage a department a supervisor must develop and continually nurture an effective communicating relationship with each employee. Such one-to-one contacts with individual employees are essential in maintaining that communicating relationship.

A CONTINUING TASK

Maintenance and improvement of the employees' channels of upward communication is a never-ending task. It must be recognized throughout that information that should be brought upward through the chain of command bears iceberg characteristics; just the tip is observed; there is always far more than meets the eye, and that which lies below the surface can be extremely damaging if ignored.

Certainly, a great deal of the information that supervisors should desire to receive from employees can be mandated through proper delegation and other direct means. However, much important and desired information will travel upward only if

- clearly recognizable means, channels, and processes are provided for employee use, and all of the available mechanisms are as nonthreatening as possible and as easy as possible for rank-and-file employees to use; and
- supervisors, higher management, and indeed the sometimes bewilderingly complex structure known to the employee as "the organization" (or perhaps as only "they") have credibility with the employees, and, through fair and consistent treatment, have earned the employees' trust.

Overcoming major barriers to true two-way communication with employees

Charles R. McConnell
Vice President for Employee Affairs
The Genesee Hospital
Rochester, New York

MOST WORKING supervisors will agree that establishing and maintaining open, two-way communication with employees is important. Many managers, however, tend to be one-way communicators, even though they well know they should try to draw employees into a two-way communication process. They readily concede the value of two-way communication but, on reflection, may also concede that active, two-way communication receives more verbal tribute than actual practice.

This article will compare one-way communication with effective two-way communication, isolate the major barriers to true two-way communication, and suggest how these barriers may be overcome (or at least their negative effects minimized).

One-way communication is a misnomer. The one-way process is not communication; it is simply the dispensing of information to another person, information that may or may not be received in the form intended. Communication might be adequately de-

Health Care Superv, 1989, 7(4), 77–82
© 1989 Aspen Publishers, Inc.

scribed as the transfer of meaning or the transfer of understanding. The objective of communication is to transfer information from the mind of one party to the mind of another in such a way that the two parties share a common meaning or a common understanding. To effect this transfer with any real assurance of success requires feedback.

In its simplest form, feedback is acknowledgment that the message has been received and understood as intended. In its more complex forms, feedback becomes part of an exchange process that eventually leads to common meaning or understanding. In any case, true communication exhibits a two-way characteristic that always includes "closing the loop" with the originator of a given message.

To understand why we frequently use the one-way process when we clearly know the two-way process is more effective, we must examine four dimensions of communication: (1) accuracy of resulting judgments, (2) interference encountered, (3) time devoted to the process, and (4) position of the sender of the message.

ACCURACY OF JUDGMENTS

Consciously pursued, two-way communication results in greater understanding or more accurate judgments than are possible with the one-way process. This fact can be repeatedly established through controlled experiments and simple exercises in an informal setting. However, knowing that transfer of meaning and understanding is appreciably greater with the two-way process than with the one-way process does not in itself make managers effective two-way communicators. On the contrary, the re-

maining three major dimensions of communication solely and together create pressures that encourage us to be one-way dispensers of information.

Most of us behave as though we believe—perhaps unconsciously—that we communicate better than we really do. People commonly blame others for communication difficulties. When you say in frustration, "The trouble with this place is there's no communication," rarely if ever are you talking about yourself.

Thus we necessarily have some difficulty imagining ourselves on a fully equal footing with those with whom we communicate. Each of us goes forward acting out in daily relationships a set of beliefs that might be described as, *"I understand what I'm saying, therefore you must understand what I'm saying because I'm a good communicator and I just gave you my understanding."*

INTERFERENCE OR "NOISE"

"Noise," a term borrowed from electronics, means exactly what the word suggests: interference or static. Noise is unwelcome in both interpersonal communication and electronics, but a certain amount of noise is inevitable.

Consider a radio. The only way to absolutely guarantee that a radio will never produce static is to turn it off and leave it that way, but doing so negates the purpose of the instrument. In interpersonal communication, the only way to guarantee the complete absence of noise is to refrain completely from interchange with others, an equally unacceptable solution.

Noise in interpersonal communication is information that is unwanted, unneeded, and, occasionally, disruptive or even destructive. Noise includes extraneous words that might be used in making a point, false starts and blind alleys encountered while trying to reach agreement between parties, the confusion arising when semantic barriers are encountered in our use of the dynamic set of symbolic tools we know as language, and the arguments and displays of temper that result when emotional barriers to communication are encountered. In short, noise is undesirable and often unpleasant, but it is a completely unavoidable part of two-way communication.

We frequently shy away from disagreement, go to great lengths to avoid confusion, and, without consciously intending to do so, drift toward one-way transfer of information because the one-way posture inhibits interchange, limits feedback, and thus discourages noise. Noise is largely unpleasant. Noise is also time consuming.

TIME

Lack of time is one of the two greatest barriers to effective two-way communication. Two-way communication transfers information more accurately than a one-way transfer, but it takes more time.

Time is a precious commodity to any serious manager. Rarely is there enough time to do everything that ought to be done, let alone time to accomplish everything as thoroughly or completely as possible. Time pressures push us toward being one-way communicators; we dispense orders or instructions in response to the needs of the moment and proceed immediately to the next issue.

The time saved when one deals with a problem quickly and "efficiently" in one-way fashion is at best a temporary gain, frequently resulting in future difficulties that require more time. Still, the temptation to yield to the pressure of time is great. Surely, not everything dealt with in quick, shoot-from-the-hip fashion will blow up and cause more trouble. Much of the time we can shoot from the hip with fairly consistent success. However, only one problem that grows to major proportions can more than negate the effects of dozens of quick fixes.

In the long run, thorough, two-way communication saves time and avoids aggravation. However, since the preferred process takes more time than might seem available, it is understandable that we frequently opt for the quickest way to satisfy the needs of the moment.

THE SENDER'S POSITION

The sender's position can be one of the two greatest barriers to true two-way communication. The sender is the originator of the message. The sender's position is his or her attitude toward the message, the recipient of the message, and the context within which the message is delivered. This total posture is governed by a combination of organization environment and authority structure, the sender's attitude toward authority and subordinates, subordinates' expectations, and the psychological makeup of the sender.

Noise is undesirable and often unpleasant, but it is a completely unavoidable part of two-way communication.

If, through some combination of factors and forces, the sender comes across as authoritarian—*"This is it, folks; I'm the boss and you're here to do what I say"*—then that sender will tend to be a one-way dispenser of orders and instructions. The strictest examples of this behavior are found in military and bureaucratic settings. Because a great deal of authoritarianism remains in many management approaches, no organization is immune to authoritarian behavior. Although most managers can be counted on to occasionally say, "My door is always open," these words often convey one message while the speakers' attitudes and behavior carry an opposite message.

Employees who expect authoritarian behavior from managers are unlikely to offer feedback or otherwise attempt to engage in a two-way process. Employees respond to the environment in which they work; if that environment discourages challenge or interchange, employees are unlikely to speak up.

Simply knowing about the barriers and acknowledging the effects they can have on your ability to communicate with employees is at least half the battle.

The sender's position may also be strongly influenced by individual psychological makeup. A sender might—entirely unconsciously—adopt a closed, one-way posture because of self-doubt, a perceived shortage of information, or a general feeling of inadequacy. In other words, the closed posture is often adopted automatically because the results are less threatening than leaving one's self open to challenge.

When operating from a one-way posture, the sender is secure, discourages feedback, and thus averts challenge, and avoids having to clarify or—the ultimate, unexpressed fear—to change anything that has already been said.

In true two-way communication, the sender is vulnerable. The sender may be challenged, may be asked to clarify, may be proven wrong, and may even be forced to abandon a starting position and adopt another view. Since few of us can ever be completely comfortable with total vulnerability, we consequently tend to withdraw within ourselves and drift toward being one-way dispensers of information.

OVERCOMING THE BARRIERS

How does one go about overcoming the barriers to effective two-way communication? Simply knowing about the barriers and acknowledging the effects they can have on your ability to communicate with employees is at least half the battle. Once an obstacle is known and understood it can be more readily recognized and avoided.

To ensure that *judgment or understanding* is accurate, accept the need for a reasonable amount of assurance that your messages are being received as intended. Take the time for a reasonable amount of interchange; perhaps nothing more is necessary than having an employee quickly restate what you said—in his or her own words. You certainly need not risk offending an employee by taking the attitude that "I want to see if you understand what I said." Rather, your approach should be that you, the sender, want to be sure you delivered the right message. If you thus look for some assurance of accuracy in each of your interpersonal transactions, you will improve the accuracy with which you transfer information overall.

Accept a certain amount of *noise* as inevitable in the process of communication. Noise seeks its own level most of the time; that is, a given amount of noise will spread itself fairly evenly throughout the two-way process in spite of anything you might do to restrict its presence. Accept noise as part of communication, but take some steps to control it. Keep your discussion on the intended topics; avoid peripheral issues and tangential conversational forays; keep social conversation to a polite minimum; and, when dealing with a group, attempt to control the gathering according to an agenda (surely Roberts' Rules of Order and other meeting-control approaches evolved at least in part to limit noise while ensuring that everyone could be heard). Appreciate that *time* now invested in two-way communication will pay for itself, perhaps several times over, in the form of time saved because future difficulties have been avoided. Conversely, appreciate that the matter dispensed summarily with now may promote misunderstanding. Such a misunderstanding can result in conditions that will take a great deal of time to correct. In the long run, true two-way communication makes more efficient use of your time.

The characteristics of the *sender's position* often represent obstacles that are among the most difficult for the individual to recognize and deal with. Much of your communications posture is adopted for reasons unknown to you and which, even if known, you would find difficult if not impossible to explain. You might, for example, project an attitude of being closed to challenge on a

certain issue. Most people can see this, but you cannot see it yourself and should someone tell you about it you might even vigorously disagree.

These small but visible signs can suggest closed posture on your part: a fleeting sense of irritation when an employee asks you to repeat seemingly simple instructions; impatience with the employee who responds to your explanation with "Yes, but what if. . ." or some similar challenge; staff meetings that are essentially your own monologues and are hurried because there is "too much of importance" to cover, allowing little time for any but the simplest questions; and thoughts like, "I'm the boss, so why should I have to put up with this from people who are supposed to be doing as I say?"

The truly effective two-way communicating manager will accept a considerable amount of vulnerability, although this is far easier said than done. The effective communicator rarely adopts a position and staunchly refuses to budge and never prohibits challenge. Rather, the effective communicator welcomes challenge with the knowledge that a sound idea can only be strengthened by challenge, and that, conversely, an idea that is weakened by challenge was probably unsound to begin with and ought to be changed.

•   •   •

True two-way communication always includes interchange, always allows for direct feedback, and occurs when one is able to avoid two major assumptions that lead to communication failure: (1) others understand what you are saying simply because you have said it (after all, *you* understand what you are saying); and (2) you understand what others are saying without seeking confirmation of your understanding. When either of these assumptions is govern-ing our behavior, interchange is lacking, we have fallen back into the one-way transfer of information, and the chances of misunderstanding are far greater than they need be.

Part III
Self-Help for the Supervisor

Improving communication: The use of management parables

Bernard L. Brown, Jr.
Executive Director
Kennestone Regional Healthcare
  System
Marietta, Georgia

COMMUNICATION. The mere mention of the term invokes a desire to insert "lack of" before it, thus creating a phrase that seems to be used more often than the word itself. "Lack of communication" currently receives the blame for everything from trouble at home to trouble on the job. It is hard to glance through a magazine or journal of any kind without being deluged with ideas for improvement in one of man's most basic areas of need: communication with others. Included are suggestions for getting a message across and, in turn, interpreting those of others; for dealing diplomatically with coworkers in stressful situations; for communicating a sense of corporate ethics to those in the work place, and on and on. Yet, one person's panacea for dealing with this modern problem could well be another's pitfall. Perhaps a "back to the

Health Care Superv, 1988, 6(2), 13–26
© 1988 Aspen Publishers, Inc.

basics" approach may be the best method to use to ensure good communication.

Ronald Reagan seems to be a master at this approach. Even those who have different political philosophies agree that he is a "Great Communicator" because of his skill in presenting information using clear, easily remembered, and readily understood methods. His secret? He makes heavy use of anecdotes and descriptive illustrations—parables, if you will—to convey messages that can help to create a strong bond with those in his audiences, most of whom can see a little of themselves in his stories.

Another man who lived long before Ronald Reagan began to make use of the parable in public speaking was Jesus. His words cut across crowds of people from every walk of life because they were presented in story form and appealed to the educated, ignorant, rich, poor, rulers, and slaves alike. People today can still identify with the concept of unconditional forgiveness illustrated in the parable of the prodigal son, for example. The son had disgraced his family and broken his father's heart by gambling his inheritance and frolicking his life away. Yet because he had a loving father, it was never too late for a second chance. The warm welcome home signified by the preparation and serving of the "fatted calf" to this wayward son is part of the language used even now in referring to the way a host welcomes guests. The fact that such stories are still meaningful more

than 1,900 years later gives proof to the fact that a good story leaves a lasting impression.

Another great teacher, Confucius, also used stories and parables to illustrate moral principles to his followers. Confucius once said, "An oppressive government is more to be feared than a tiger." A mental picture of that grasping, growling tiger of a government could easily be captured in a political cartoon today—never to be forgotten.

Storytellers down through the ages have captivated audiences from small groups around the campfire to great crowds in arenas. Nothing can quiet a group of children like the promise of a story and when a story is told to drive home a point, chances are the teller will not be disappointed in the results.

But what does this have to do with communication in management? Is there value in this back-to-the-basics, homespun approach of using parables and stories to communicate for the modern health care supervisor?

The executive director of a 650-bed hospital system in Georgia says there is. He believes that by adapting these time-proven methods of instilling ideas, managers can communicate clearly such concepts as commitment to service, excellence of performance, and personal involvement to those with whom they work. Going a step further, there is little doubt that an organization that effectively instills these ideals throughout its ranks will be a worthy competitor in today's marketplace.

Where did it all begin for this chief executive and his use of management parables as a method of communication? Regularly distributed to employees is the organizational in-house newsletter. Along with the news of who was promoted, took a sabbatical, or recently joined the organization, an opportunity exists to use this forum for illustrating and underscoring corporate values. What is going to be read, remembered, and discussed? Chances are it will not be a chart or list of statistical data. A story involving someone known to readers or relating to an area of com-

---

A story involving someone known to the readers or relating to an area of common interest will probably have the most impact.

---

mon interest will probably have the most impact. Add a touch of humor or pathos, and the success of the communication is assured.

A monthly column entitled "It Seems to Me . . ." is published in *THE INNERVIEW*, the monthly newsletter of the Kennestone Regional Healthcare System. It has become a tool for this hospital administrator as he seeks to share his thoughts and feelings about the challenges of working in a large hospital system. Over the past 16 years, he has established a rapport with employees, physicians, patients, and other readers from all over the area by sim-

ply "telling it like it is" in down-home style.

How does it work? Certain monthly columns speak for themselves in communicating the desirability of commitment to service, excellence of performance, and personal involvement. Reader comment has given credence to the hope that the message has come through loud and clear. The "story" makes it happen.

BE COMMITTED TO SERVICE

For employees in the health care field, and perhaps especially in hospitals, a commitment to service is paramount. The manager who can communicate the importance of this through words and deeds is worthy of his or her calling; and the employee who accepts this commitment makes the circle complete. "Professionally We Serve, Personally We Care," is the motto for this particular hospital system, so the idea certainly is not new to those who work here. A case in point:

Several weeks ago, I learned unexpectedly that my brother had been in a serious automobile accident. He was conscious when he arrived in our emergency department, but was very irritable and combative before they rushed him to surgery. He must have suffered a head injury, I thought. "Did you treat him well? He's my brother," I anxiously exclaimed to the emergency department secretary.

I called surgery to make sure that the anesthesiologist and surgeon knew he was my brother. "He's special; do your best," I told the recovery room nurse. "Take good care of him. He's my brother."

About the time he was to go to the intensive care unit, I was called into an important committee meeting. As the session dragged on, all I could think about was my brother upstairs in critical condition. I stepped out for a moment and called the unit. "Give him the best nursing care available; he's my brother," I frantically requested.

They kept him in isolation overnight because there was risk of infection. I asked the evening supervisor to make certain that he was comfortable and well-cared for. "He's my brother," I told her. I hardly slept that night. I prayed that he would recover completely.

Even though I have worked in a hospital for many years now, sometimes it seems impersonal. I often get bogged down in day-to-day activities and I forget that we are treating people, real people. I sometimes even forget that our true purpose is to *professionally serve and personally care.* But when my brother came into our hospital, I immediately regained my perspective and our sense of purpose became very clear to me.

As I walked in the door the next morning, I was told that my brother was out of danger and had been transferred to a regular nursing unit. I could visit him for the first time. Before going up, I called every department that had served him to thank them for taking such good care of my brother. Interestingly, most had not realized that he was the brother of the administrator because his last name was different from mine. They were just doing the usual good job of serving and caring, which they always do.

It seems to me that this is what a hospital is all about. Special care rendered by special people to patients who are very

special to folks like me. In other words, serving our brothers.

Since I was the only boy born into the Brown family, I guess I was just thinking that all men are my brothers.[1]

HOW TO SERVE DIFFICULT PATIENTS

Making an initial commitment to serve is only the first step. What happens when the going gets rough and the very ones who need serving are not so easy to serve?

I have a 16-year-old son, and he is one of the greatest joys of my life. He is not full-grown yet, but he can already beat me on the tennis court (most of the time), and can slam-dunk a basketball on our backyard goal, which we have lowered from regulation height. (Incidentally, in a recent game of one-on-one, I just about broke my back trying to dunk it myself.) And he makes decent grades, too. But if you have ever had a teenage boy, you know it ain't all "good." At times, he can be rude, self-centered, and even downright ornery. Even though I love him more than most everything in life, I often find myself not liking him very much because of his behavior and manners. However, from conferences on raising teenagers, conversations with other parents, and even from my own experience, I have learned that he is just as normal as apple pie. During the period when a boy is passing from childhood through adolescence into manhood, he is just not very easy to get along with. He can drive you up the wall, and many times you really have to work at liking him.

I bring this up primarily because I have noticed that there is another group of individuals who are also not very likeable at times. I do not know about you, but I find that many patients are hard to get along with. They are hurting, they are often mad, they are very demanding, they are preoccupied with their own problems, and in general, they are just not in a good frame of mind. All of these and other traits just make them poor candidates for most likeable among our acquaintances.

As health care professionals charged with the responsibility of serving these sometimes unlikeable people, how do we deal with our tendency to strike back, respond negatively, or to be apathetic about their needs? It seems to me that the situation here is similar to the one that I have in my relationship with my son. If that be the case, we need to look at it from the same perspective.

We must realize that people who are usually quite amiable may become self-centered, demanding, and even obnoxious during the times they are patients in an alien setting like a hospital. Most are going through a dramatic and often critical event in their lives. To hospital workers, this can be a source of great frustration or it can be the opportunity for greatest satisfaction, depending upon how we respond. Anyone can love the likeable, but only special people can love the unlikeable. It is the nature of hospital folks to love the latter, perhaps in the same way that a father loves his teenage son.

I am confident that my son will be president of the United States in about 30 years if he wants to be, provided that I don't do away with him before he's 17.[2]

GO THE SECOND MILE

And then there is the "going the second mile" concept that comes nat-

urally for a few, but needs to be "driven home" to most. Those consumers of the services rendered by health care workers *may* remember the good treatment they received as part of the job; but they will *never* forget the little extras that those same folks extended to them simply because they cared.

I learned of an incident several weeks ago that impressed me tremendously.

While waiting in front of the hospital for her ride, one of our employees noticed another lady walking back and forth with a worried look on her face. Our lady inquired, "Is there something I can help you with?" This opened a conversation that lasted for several minutes.

It seemed that the visitor was from an adjoining state. Her 22-year-old son had been in a bad automobile accident and was to be hospitalized here for several more weeks. She needed to return to her job back home, but also felt that she should stay. Our employee got the lady's name and the room number of her son.

The next day, she visited the young man and his mother, and because of her warm, caring manner, they became friends immediately. As she left that day our lady said, "If you need to go on home, why don't you let me check on your son every day and if he needs anything, I'll let you know. Also, if you get concerned, just call me and I will take care of whatever is needed."

The grateful mother went home assured that everything would be all right and returned several weeks later to pick up her son. Incidentally our lady has a son about the same age. The thank you note from the grateful mother was beautiful.

It seems to me that this is what "Personally We Care" is all about.[3]

COMMUNICATE BY PRECEPT AND EXAMPLE

An administrator, manager, or supervisor can also communicate through deeds—by precept and ex-

---

An administrator, manager, or supervisor can also communicate through deeds—by precept and example, to be specific.

---

ample, to be specific. This method of communication becomes even more effective when he or she can admit mistakes and show growth and maturity in a certain area as a result. It may sound strange, but the idea of servitude begins *at the top* in a service-oriented organization; the top sets the tone that others will follow.

As part of my presentation to new employees at the biweekly orientation program, I talk about our philosophy of serving. I usually make note of the fact that a hospital is a service organization that provides a service that, generally, people would rather do without. This fact leads us to the conclusion that we, as individuals working in a hospital setting, must be servants to others if our institution is to fulfill its true purpose.

This philosophy had always sounded good and moral, and the purpose of its inclusion in my orientation speech was to inspire and motivate our new personnel. However, this idea had been somewhat remote to me personally because I had become isolated and insulated from its demands while working in my big, plush office, among executive types and with

most of my time occupied with "important" meetings and conferences.

However, I regained my perspective one day during an interview when a young man asked me to define the title, "Administrator." I proceeded to expound upon my virtues as a leader, the many significant duties that I perform and climaxed the definition with the power and prestige I enjoy. Then he asked, "From where is the word administrator derived?" According to my dictionary, I discovered the base or root word is minister, which means to serve. This revelation humbled me and caused me to feel hypocritical but, at the same time, it seemed to me that the words hospital and administrator fit together better than I had ever noticed before. A service organization needs to be headed by a serving leader.[4]

ACHIEVE EXCELLENCE OF PERFORMANCE

Not only must health care employees serve, they must strive to serve *well*. Excellence of performance at every level of an organization ensures its success as a whole. Every position is important or it would not exist, and all employees need to be reminded of their importance from the first day on the job. The wise supervisor will inspire and challenge his or her workers to attain high goals despite weaknesses and obstacles that sometimes work against them.

A memorable story about a trained chicken in a Soviet circus brought a warm response from the father of a retarded employee, expressing his appreciation for an organization that allowed his son to use the talents that he had and to develop new ones that no one suspected. This father wrote, "Bill never accepted (his disabilities) as a reason for not attempting to live a normal life. We're very proud of Bill and hope you are proud to have him on your staff."

A couple of years ago, I had the privilege of traveling in the Soviet Union with a group of hospital administrators who were observing the health care system in that country. Even though this was the opportunity of a lifetime, I find that I can remember less and less about my experiences there as time goes by. Then periodically something triggers my memory about certain places or things and it all comes back to me. For example, the recent miniseries on Peter the Great reminded me of our visit to Leningrad.

Those of you who know me personally recognize that I am not the most intellectual or perceptive individual in the world. Therefore, I tend to relate to the very basic, simple things in life. The reason I mention this is that I saw something the other day that carried me back to my Soviet tour.

While driving in a rural area of the "promised land" (South Georgia) on my way to join my hunting partner, I rode by a farmhouse and saw a chicken walking along the edge of a fence like it was on a tightrope. This reminded me of a visit to the world-famous Moscow Circus. Here, in a traditional roundtop tent, I saw one of the greatest circus performances you could imagine. You will not believe this, but one of the star attractions was a trained chicken. In pure amazement, I watched that chicken ride a bike, count, dance, sing, and do things I have only seen trained dogs, lions, tigers, and bears do.

I guess the reason this seemed so astonishing was that I never imagined a chicken could do such things. This was totally out of character. In my mind, chickens were only good for eggs and frying.

It seems to me that there are some folks around who are much like that trained chicken. We never dreamed they could be trained to do anything. We never expected them to accomplish so much. Surely, success in their field of endeavor was not expected.

I still can't believe a little five-foot-seven-inch tall basketball player won the National Basketball Association's slam-dunk contest. The Atlanta Hawk guard, Spud Webb, is even more amazing to me than that Moscow Circus chicken.

Some of the other "trained chickens" of the world include: a deaf composer—Ludwig van Beethoven, a "retarded learner"—Albert Einstein, a blind musician—Ray Charles, a "too old" painter—Grandma Moses, a victim of racial prejudice—George Washington Carver, and a multiple amputee—Max Cleland, former head of the Veterans Administration.

Most of us tend to conform ourselves to society's expectations instead of venturing a bit out of character toward something special and unique. It seems to me that doing our thing in life's center ring is far better than just waiting to be plucked.[5]

USE HUMOR AS A COMMUNICATION TOOL

Never underestimate the power of humor as a communication tool. Like a spoonful of sugar, it makes the medicine go down easily. If the joke is on oneself, the points made are even easier to take. The next anecdote catches the writer in the act of being human, reveals him to be as prone to error as the next person, but also encourages the reader to recognize faults and to strive on toward excellence.

One of my very best friends tells the story about an experience he and I had when we were teenagers. Of course he embellishes and exaggerates this yarn a bit, but here is my version.

While fishing one day, I found a "fly" (small artificial lure) on an overhanging limb at the edge of the pond. Evidently another fisherman had lost it earlier. The fly was in good shape, so I stuck it on my shirt collar for safekeeping.

As we finished fishing at the end of the day and were paddling the boat toward shore, my friend noticed a "bug" on my collar. He shouted, "There's a bee on your shirt!" I could see its wings through the corner of my eye, so I started slapping the "bee." Of course this was the fly that I had rescued from the limb. Each time I hit it with my hand, the hook stuck in my shoulder, which felt like a bee sting. My only hope to rid myself of this killer bee was to go overboard, which I proceeded to do. It was only after I was soaked to the gills that I remembered placing the fly on my collar.

What's the point in telling this humorous story? Maybe there are a few lessons here. First, we tend to have lapses in memory; second, artificial replicas often look like the real thing; and third, we sometimes react drastically without having all the facts. Certainly these are natural human traits, but interestingly, we need to counteract all three tendencies as we function as health care professionals.

Let's take these one at a time. To forget something important relative to a pa-

tient's care can have serious consequences. Therefore, documentation is crucial. To fail to distinguish between genuine medical clues and facsimiles can lead to misdiagnosis and faulty treatment practices. And finally, to act from an emotional rather than a factual standpoint almost always produces less than desirable results. In summary, *recording our actions, discovering the facts, and acting appropriately based on these facts* should be standard procedure in any health care institution. These three rules help us to overcome our human tendencies toward forgetfulness, laxness, and indiscriminate reaction.

You know, life might be awfully boring and mundane if we had the capacity to remember everything, to see everything clearly, and to act appropriately in every case—in other words, to be perfect. It seems to me a more realistic challenge is to recognize our human frailties and take appropriate steps to overcome our weaknesses.

To consider ourselves perfect is the height of human vanity; to be effective despite our imperfections is the epitome of human achievement.[6]

BLOOM WHERE YOU ARE PLANTED

"Bloom where you are planted" is a sound piece of advice, for it implies that anyone can reach a degree of excellence in life, regardless of his or her positioning on life's scale. A job that may be ideally suited to one person's talents may be totally wrong for another. Yet, when all are planted in the right "row" in an organizational "garden" the end result can be very effective. This can never be stressed too much when communicating organizational values to employees.

All of us have qualities and talents that are uniquely our own, but I am sure that there is not one of us who has not wanted to be just like someone else in one way or another. It is what we perceive as our weaknesses that we want to change, but sometimes those weaknesses are really strengths in disguise. Let me give you an example.

I may be the world's best sidewalk superintendent because I love building programs and really enjoy watching them during the different stages of construction. The other day, I was out observing the progress on the physicians' parking deck. It was a hot, busy day out there. Forms were being erected, decking and pans were being put into place, and two concrete trucks were waiting to pour. There must have been 25 workmen busy as bees preparing the upper level for concrete. Most of these guys (no women were on this crew) had on tank tops or no shirts at all. You could tell they were all in great shape; many were downright musclebound.

But one fellow seemed out of place in this setting. He was probably a foot shorter than any of the others and lacked all the protruding muscles. Because he was so conspicuously different, I remember thinking to myself, "I wonder how that little guy got a construction job?"

Then I saw why he was there. The foreman called him over. Evidently, inside the forms for a main column, the supporting steel rods or some part of the interior framing had slipped out of place. The choices to remedy the situation seemed to be either take all the forms apart or have someone go down in this 18-inch hollow square form to correct the problem. This little guy was the only person small enough to fit. Five minutes later, he emerged the hero who had saved the day, and the work continued on schedule.

After watching all of this, I have concluded that maybe success should be measured not so much by our physical attributes, our mental capabilities, or even our spiritual maturity, as by the weaknesses and limitations that we have overcome while striving to succeed. These, rather than the things which come easy, tend to extract the best that is in us.

A little fellow, who would have probably preferred to be larger and taller, could do something no one else could do, and as a result, all benefited from his special traits. He turned his weakness into a strength.

To want to be like someone else is a human tendency; to desire to be unique and special is the result of a divine revelation.[7]

DARE TO BE DIFFERENT

Speaking of blooming, there are always those who bloom a little longer, shine a little brighter, or strive a little harder in their quest for success in the work place. These people may not be any smarter or have any more talent than others around them, but they dare to be different, to reach outside their immediate grasp, to stretch, grow, and improve. A story about one of the South's most beautiful flowers, the azalea, communicates this ideal.

This spring has been one of the most beautiful in a long time; probably because we had so much rain. The azaleas were particularly gorgeous this year.

While walking up the front sidewalk a

few weeks ago, I noticed a single azalea bush next to the building that had three different colors of flowers on it. One was white, another was a light pink, and the third was a deeper, reddish color. I observed it every day until the petals fell off, and to me it was the prettiest plant in the bed. I started asking some of my horticultural and plant-growing friends about this interesting phenomenon. It amazed them, too. One suggested that the bees must have gotten mixed up when passing the pollen around.

Now what is the moral of this little story? It probably does not really have one. But it seems to me (an old philosophical romantic) that sometimes being different can be beautiful. To go along with the crowd, to conform, to blend, is generally safe; but to dare to be different, to try new ways, to explore different approaches, can make one stand out. We have some of these conspicuously unique individuals in our organization, and they help make our hospital even better as they work beside us every day. Thank God for all types that make an organization great.[8]

USE THE PERSONAL TOUCH

It is difficult to do well as a worker in the health care field without some degree of personal involvement. The very nature of the job demands it, in fact, for "serving" is a lonely experience if "caring" is missing. This is not to say that an employee must shoulder the burden of each case; there are not enough hours in the day for that. However, at the time in which he or she is directly involved

with another person, be it patient, visitor, or fellow employee, the "personal touch" is a necessity.

As in serving and striving for excellence of performance, personal involvement must begin at the top. A manager who cares enough to show feelings spreads the message that it is

---

A manager who cares enough to show feelings spreads the message that it is okay, and rises quite a few steps in the eyes of those who are watching and listening.

---

okay, and rises quite a few steps in the eyes of those who are watching and listening. This administrator learned a valuable lesson in the face of the adversity going on around him and shared it in a very human way.

I cried the other day. I closed the door to my office and actually cried. This emotional outburst was the result of three visits with patients and/or members of their families. I know these folks personally and each of them is considered part of our hospital family because of their involvement with the volunteer program. All three have cancer.

The first is a volunteer who has been fighting this disease for more than 15 years. She has been an inspiration to me and has helped numerous other patients suffering from the same illness. She had tears in her eyes as we talked about her involvement at the hospital. She did not know what the immediate future held, but I could sense a peace about her during my visit.

The second was another volunteer who grows some of the most beautiful roses I have ever seen. During our conversation, she told me about how her doctor had broken the news to the family about her disease. She shared with me the fact that she was not concerned about herself, but instead she was worried about her "boys" because they were so worried about her. I noticed sadness in her face as she told me all this, but there was also a certain inner peace about her.

Then I stopped by to see the son of one of our newer volunteers. He is a college student and an outstanding young man. Due to the disease he had lost a leg earlier and was again in a battle due to recurring tumors. We talked for a long time, and during the course of the conversation he mentioned several of our employees, by name, who had given him such loving care.

I share these three experiences with you because I learned something significant that day. I have always been told that doctors, nurses, and other hospital people are supposed to refrain from becoming emotionally involved with patients because it makes our jobs too hard. We are not supposed to cry. However, after thinking about this a great deal, it seems to me that there is nothing wrong with crying. It would be hard to really care for folks if you could not cry with them.

I did not know that day what the future held for these three special people, and to be honest, I do not know what the future holds for any of us. However, I do know after three visits that I had a hard time making, I felt a peace myself. I went to give, but I received.

On second thought, I do know what the ultimate future holds. I hope you do, too.[9]

GET INVOLVED

All great organizations have exceptional employees who get *involved* day after day. Sometimes they are behind the scenes and at times out in front, taking time to care and to let others know that they do. In one situation, this all came together at the funeral of a faithful, long-term security officer for the hospital system.

From time to time, situations arise that remind me how much I appreciate the excellent board of trustees, medical and administrative staffs, and volunteers we have in our organization. However, daily, and even hourly, incidents come to my attention that make me realize how thankful I am for the great employees we have working at our hospital. I could probably write a book about hospital employees, but let me just mention one as a "for instance."

Right before Christmas, I attended the funeral of a good man and a true friend. The preacher, while giving the eulogy, made the observation that probably all those in attendance had been helped by this man in finding a parking place at the hospital. Most smiled and acknowledged that this was true. Family and friends of patients at this large, busy hospital come and go constantly and most had been greeted by this friendly gentleman who had only one good eye. Fred worked as a security officer for almost 16 years here after a long career with the U.S. Postal Service. As best we could determine from our files, he held the record (12 years) for not missing a single day's work, reporting to work late, or leaving work early.

I did not realize Fred's impact on our

organization until several years ago. While attending a meeting, I was introduced to a prominent individual whom I had never met before. Of course, being the chief executive officer of one of the largest institutions in our community, I was braced to acknowledge the admiration and accolades that I anticipated from this person for my achievements. However, when he learned where I worked, his face lit up and he exclaimed, "That's great, you work at Fred's hospital."

That's right, I work at Fred's hospital. I also work at Janie's, Gloria's, Linda's, Myrtle's, Ursula's, Lisa's, Shirley's, Dorothy's, Emily's, Bobbie's, Peter's, Rene's, Vi's, Sharon's, Carolyn's, Jennelle's, Claire's, Charlie's, Marcia's, Ann's, Len's, Grace's, Sara's, Beverly's, Tony's, Debra's, Buddy's, Pearl's, Tom's, Janet's, Sandi's, Carol's, Cathy's, Sherrie's, Barry's, Greg's, Jane's, Joe's, Denyse's, Louise's, Linda's, Jimmy's, Betty's, Freda's, Mary Jane's, Barbara's, Kaye's, Mary Ann's, Donna's, Saundra's, Jeanne's, John's, Alta's, Toni's, and Anne's . . . hospital, too!

It seems to me that a hospital is only as good as its employees and that is why this one is a great institution. Because I knew Fred personally, there is no doubt in my mind that he is helping folks find a parking place up in Heaven right now. I just hope that it's as crowded there as it is in our parking lot![10]

Physicians, nurses, and others in direct contact with patients probably have the worst time of all in knowing how far to go with "personal involvement." After all, they deal daily with the sick and dying. How do they stand it? Wouldn't it be better to remain cold and remote to protect themselves from constant emotional pain? This administrator says, "No way," and has seen just the opposite over and over in his organization.

A close friend of mine was recently hospitalized for several weeks on 6 North. As I went to see him each day, I decided to get some exercise by walking up the stairs to the sixth floor. It was very tough the first few days, but got better as time passed. Not only did this daily ritual help my body, but it also lifted my spirits. Let me share one of my experiences in the stairwell.

On one particular day, I met one of our physicians and an employee coming down the steps. The employee was crying and the doctor was attempting to console her. My first thought was that I had intruded into a personal matter, but then the doctor said, "We're both upset because we just lost one of our patients." I knew both these individuals' professional capabilities were outstanding, but I had never seen their hearts exposed like this before. They were using the stairwell as a sort of haven where they could let their feelings show. As I passed, I thought to myself, "That's the kind of folks I want to care for me when I'm sick."

Joseph Cardinal Bernadin, in a speech delivered to the Congress on Administration, Chicago, Illinois, February 1984, said it beautifully: "We have as our core vocation the task of providing caring and careful service to our brothers and sisters in the human family. See how these health care professionals love one another. See how caring and careful they are, in their efforts to serve the human family. See how wondrous is their task. See how dedicated is their service. See how skillful is their effort."

My friend has gone home from the hospital, but I still walk up to the top floor every day. It is amazing what we discover in the most unlikely places.[11]

WORK TOGETHER

Communication about personal involvement would not mean a thing if the people working together were not doing just that—working together. *Esprit de corps* is a term that has come to the forefront to describe a healthy environment in the work place where employees care about one another and about the future and success of their organization. This family-type concept was pointed out quite clearly during a hospital blood drive.

The Red Cross bloodmobile was here in the hospital recently and I went by to donate my blood. Usually around 9:00 A.M. the initial crowd has cleared, but in this instance, the line was backed up down the corridor all the way to the cafeteria. I had a meeting at 10:00 A.M., so I knew that I wouldn't have time to be processed. I returned after lunch, but found a similar situation, and then again during the middle of the afternoon the line was still very long. Finally, at 6:30 that evening, they finished taking my blood. I was the next to last of 282 who gave that day. This was a one-day record for us that may never be broken. Normally, 150 units is considered excellent.

What made this particular blood drive different from all the others? A few weeks earlier, the son of one of our best nurses was injured in a near-fatal accident at a construction site. As a consequence, David lost a leg, had multiple operations, and will require extensive therapy over the next few months. In the course of his treatment, he had received around 95 units of blood. Thank goodness he has come a long, long way so far, and will continue to improve.

The Red Cross had publicized the fact that they were short of blood at this time of year, but more significant in this case, word had spread that one of our hospital family needed blood. In addition to our folks, people from David's church, Dobbins Air Force Base where his father works, and Lockheed, the employer of one of his aunt's, contributed greatly to the success of this drive.

More important than the record number of donors, many individuals gave blood for the first time. Several had to overcome great fear of the needle. I even saw several doctors donating their blood.

This particular blood drive by all accounts was special. It seems to me that it was special to most of us who participated because it was personal. When things get personal with us, our spirits rise and what before was considered an obligation becomes a privilege.

I signed my name to David's get-well card while I was drinking three cups of fruit juice and eating more than my share of peanut butter cookies. Then I left immediately to attend the monthly Utilization Review Committee meeting. I was back in the real world of the hospital business, but for those few minutes while my blood was being pumped out, I thought to myself, "This is what we are really here for." Professionally We Serve, Personally We Care.[12]

•   •   •

It is amazing how stories in a monthly column can communicate such high ideals as commitment to service, excellence of performance and personal involvement over and over again to the readers. Some of those parables will never be forgotten because they touched a familiar chord, brought back a memory, or helped solve a problem in a person's life. At other times, readers may be encouraged to reach for goals they never knew possible simply because someone else in a similar situation proved they were obtainable.

Never underestimate the power of a parable or story. Storytelling has been a part of human life since time began. If a sophisticated organization like a modern hospital can learn from such a down-home method of communication, it will be around for years to come.

REFERENCES

1. "My Brother's Keeper." *The Innerview*, 4, no. 9, June 1986, p. 4.
2. Brown, Jr., B. L., *Professionally We Serve, Personally We Care*. Columbus, Ga: Quill Publications, 1985, pp 88–89.
3. Ibid.
4. Ibid.
5. "The Trained Chicken." *The Innerview*, 4, no. 8, 1986, p. 4.
6. "The Lure of the Killer Bee." *The Innerview*, 5, no. 1, 1986, p. 4.
7. "Finding a Perfect Fit." *The Innerview*, 3, no. 12, 1985.
8. Brown, *Professionally We Serve, Personally We Care*.
9. "I Cried." *The Innerview*, 3, no. 11, 1985, p. 6.
10. "Fred's Hospital." *The Innerview*, 3, no. 7, 1985, p. 4.
11. Brown, *Professionally We Serve, Personally We Care*.
12. "When David Needed Blood." *The Innerview*, 3, no. 3, 1984, p. 4.

The supervisor as a responsible listener

Harry E. Munn, Jr.
Associate Professor
Department of Speech
  Communication
North Carolina State University
Raleigh, North Carolina

G OOD LISTENING habits are
not the easiest skills to develop, and that may be why many people listen poorly. Too many times
people develop mental sets or preconceived ideas as to what is being
said. They hear the other person, but
they are not listening. Often they
miss the *real* message. They fail to
recognize the feelings that are not being articulated by words; they are not
actively involved in what is being
said. The following story illustrates
the point:

A Marine Corps general was visiting an
installation and asked to see the bugler
privately. "Can you play fire call?" he inquired.
  "Yes sir," replied the marine.
  "Then meet me tomorrow at 5:00 A.M. in
front of the post headquarters and don't
mention this to anyone," said the general.
  The post commander was so eager to

Health Care Superv, 1982,1(1),62–71
© 1982 Aspen Publishers, Inc.

know what was going on that he pressured the bugler into telling him about his conversation with the general. That night the post's fire station was a beehive of activity as equipment was washed and polished. Even the door hinges were oiled. The next morning the marine bugler reported to the general.

"Sound church call," the general ordered.

"But, sir, you asked me if I knew fire call."

"Yes, son, I know, but now please play church call."

As the first notes pierced the early morning stillness, the doors of the fire station flew open and out roared the trucks with bells clanging and sirens screaming.

Being a good listener requires intense concentration. Research has shown that people involved in active listening show degrees of tension as they try empathically to understand what has been said.

Real listening requires an expenditure of energy in obtaining and retaining the spoken discourse of others. Tests in the physiological psychology laboratory have shown that active listening demands as much energy, makes a person just as tired, as comparable efforts in speaking, reading, or writing.[1]

Research in both business and education has demonstrated that most individuals can improve in listening performance. Warren Ganong of the Methods Engineering Council compared trainees who had knowledge of listening skills to those who had no knowledge. Those with listening skill knowledge achieved marks 12 to 15 percent higher than those with no such knowledge.[2] Listening can mean greater efficiency; it stems from the need to gather necessary data. Listening helps in settling grievances. Listening makes people feel special.

Although in the form of "self-talk," sometimes referred to as intrapersonal communication, people spend a great deal of time listening to themselves, at times they do not even do that well. About 70 percent of an average working day is spent in verbal communication. Research shows that average working adults divide their communications time roughly along these lines: listening, 45 percent; talking, 30 percent; reading, 16 percent; writing, 9 percent.[3]

These statistics indicate that almost one-half of adult communication time is spent in listening. A failure to listen not only affects the relationships between health care coworkers and supervisors but also the quality of the care given to patients.

The simple test shown in the box will allow readers to rate themselves as listeners. It will also call attention to some of the skills needed to be a good listener and to some behavior that can interfere with good listening.

LISTENING FOR THE NONVERBAL MESSAGES

A good listener should begin by facing the speaker to ensure that he or she can physically hear. The listener thereby tells the sender that he or she is ready to listen, able to hear

How Do You Rate as a Listener?

Take the following test and see how you rate as a listener. Place an X in the appropriate blank. When speaking interpersonally with a coworker, patient, physician, supervisor or employee, do you:

Usually   Sometimes   Seldom

(1) Prepare yourself physically by standing or sitting, facing the speaker and making sure you can hear?

(2) Watch the speaker for the verbal as well as the nonverbal messages?

(3) Decide from the speaker's appearance and delivery whether or not what he or she has to say is worthwhile?

(4) Listen primarily for ideas and underlying feelings?

(5) Determine your own bias, if any, and try to allow for it?

(6) Keep your mind on what the speaker is saying?

(7) Interrupt immediately if you hear a statement that you feel is wrong?

(8) Try to see the situation from the other person's point of view?

(9) Try to have the last word?

(10) Make a conscientious effort to evaluate the logic and credibility of what you hear?

Scoring: This checklist, although by no means complete, should help you measure your listening ability. Score yourself as follows: Questions 1, 2, 4, 5, 6, 8 and 10—ten points for *usually,* five points for *sometimes* and zero points for *seldom.* Questions 3, 7 and 9—zero points for *usually,* five points for *sometimes* and ten points for *seldom.*

If you scored below 70, your listening skills can be improved because you have developed some undesirable listening habits. If you scored between 70 and 85, you listen well but can still improve. If you scored 90 or above, you are an excellent listener.

the verbal messages and see the nonverbal messages the speaker is sending.

People should learn to listen for the speaker's nonverbal as well as verbal messages. Everyone sends two messages. One message is sent verbally, and the other is sent nonverbally through bodily action, gestures, paralanguage (inflection in the voice) and facial expressions. The nonverbal message conveys the speaker's attitude and degree of sincerity. To miss the nonverbal message is to miss half or more of what is being said.

One message is sent verbally, and the other is sent nonverbally through bodily action, gestures, paralanguage (inflection in the voice) and facial expressions.

Facial expressions

Face-to-face attention shows that a person is interested in what is being said. People tend to avoid and look away from people and things in which they are not interested. Attention and interest are synonymous. People face and pay attention to the things they are interested in, and they are interested in the things they are facing and paying attention to.

More than 100 years ago, Charles Darwin wrote *The Expression of Emotions in Man and Animals*, the product of a century-old pursuit and one of the first works on facial expressions.[4] Darwin theorized that facial expressions are instinctive and not learned behavior. However, today most anthropologists believe that facial expressions are a result of natural reactions in the muscles and nerves of the face and of cultural conditioning that governs the expression of emotion.

In American culture, facial expressions play an important role in the social communication between people. Facial expressions can convey true feelings and be useful communicative tools. Unfortunately, however, the general rule regarding facial expressions in America seems at times to parallel that of the ancient Greek Stoics, in that Americans are taught from early childhood to avoid excessive expressive behavior, facial or otherwise. They are taught to show neutrality when angry, especially in public places. If unhappy, they are urged to show only the slightest sense of sadness in their demeanor. In this culture, as in many others, false facial expressions can be masks behind which people hide.

However, even with these limitations, the face is one of the most reliable of all nonverbal indicators. Knapp points to the importance of the face when he states, "The face is rich in communicative potential. It is the primary site for communication of emotional states; it reflects interpersonal attitudes; it provides nonverbal feedback on the comments of others; and some say it is the primary source of information next to human speech."[5]

There are six basic facial expressions: disgust, surprise, happiness, anger, sadness and fear. Several of these expressions can be exhibited at the same time. For example, an employee can simultaneously exhibit surprise and disgust or surprise and happiness.

The problem of interpretation is compounded when the verbal message seems to be in conflict with the facial expression. Most nonverbal theorists agree that if the meaning of the facial expression is clear and the verbal context in which it occurs is not clear, the face will be the most reliable source of information.

Ekman, Friesen and Ellsworth conducted an in-depth analysis of all the important studies of facial expression and concluded, "Contrary to the impressions conveyed in previous reviews of the literature that the evidence in the field is confusing and contradictory, our reanalysis showed consistent evidence of accurate judgment of emotion from facial behavior."[6] Mehrabian and Weiner found that when exposed to an inconsistent message, facial expression has the greatest impact, paralanguage (voice inflection) has the second greatest impact and verbal expression has the least impact.[7]

Eye contact

A look is more than just seeing. Meaning is constantly conveyed in numerous visual ways—through the stern look of a boss, the loving look of a patient's relative or the cooperative look of a coworker. As early as 1921, Simmel reported:

The union and interaction of individuals is based upon mutual glances. . . . By the glance which reveals the other, one discloses himself. . . . The eye cannot take unless at the same time it gives.[8]

Argyle believes there are several implicit rules about interacting visually, including:

- There is more mutual eye contact between friends than others, and a looker's frank gaze is widely interpreted as positive regard.
- Persons who seek eye contact while speaking are regarded as not only exceptionally well-disposed by their target, but also as more believable and earnest.[9]

Eye contact tells people how they are doing and the kind of relationship they have with another person. People tend to look at things they like and to look away from things they dislike. Argyle and Dean discovered that a speaker's eye contact occurs at the end of phrases and sentences but does not occur during long statements. When two people like one another, they establish eye contact more often and for longer duration than when there is dislike or tension in the relationship.[10]

Paralanguage

It has often been said by college debaters that it is not what one says that counts but how one says it. The tone of the voice conveys different types of meaning. Telephone conversations, for example, rely heavily on paralanguage. The inflection in the voice, the pauses and the rate of speech can convey anger, happiness, boredom, interest, love, hate, frustration or uncertainty. Telephone conversations do not allow people the luxury of seeing gestures, bodily actions or expressions. However, from paralanguage they attempt to visualize these nonverbal actions.

During interpersonal communication with employees, as supervisors attempt to listen, they rely heavily on paralanguage to determine the genuineness of the message. Myers and Myers cite the following examples of verbal statements and what they might really mean, depending on the paralanguage that is being used:

- Verbal: "I'll be happy to do it." Paralanguage: "I'll do it, but it will be the last time."
- Verbal: "You always make me do what you want." Paralanguage: "All right, you win."
- Verbal: "Don't worry, I'll take care of it." Paralanguage: "You're so dumb I better take care of it."[11]

HABITS OF A GOOD LISTENER

A listener should *not* decide from the speaker's appearance or delivery that what he or she has to say is worthwhile. To focus on the speaker's delivery or appearance is to become distracted from the purpose of communication: receiving the speaker's ideas. One should be more interested in what people have to say than how they say it or what they look like. One should listen for ideas and underlying feelings. Again, the purpose of good communication is to be able to reflect on and exchange ideas.

A good listener should try to determine his or her own biases, if any, and allow for them. Communication gets blamed for many things. Whenever something does not go right, it may be said that there is a communication breakdown. However, many times there is not a communication breakdown at all. In fact, communication might be very good; both parties may know what has been said, and there may be a common understanding. The parties may simply dislike what they have heard. If the health care supervisor or employee could learn to recognize such differences, better relationships would be formed. One will not always agree with everyone. The trauma in such situations develops when people discover they are no longer talking about the issues but about each other.

A good listener should attempt to keep his or her mind on what the speaker is saying. Too many times people pretend attention and, like the little dog in the back of a car window, just keep nodding their heads up and down without hearing a word of what is being said. One should *not* interrupt immediately if one hears a statement that one feels is wrong. Indeed, if one listens closely, one may be persuaded that the statement is right. Sometimes a person may fail to listen just because of this fear of something different, of the possibility that he or she may have to forsake some sacred position held for years.

A good listener should try to see the situation from the other person's point of view. Agreement is not always necessary. However, there is no way to change other people's perceptions until one can see how they have formulated those perceptions. One should *not* try to have the last word. One should listen to what is being said and then think about it. This reflection may take some time, but a person needs time to think before communicating. Sometimes, to solve the problem, a person has to walk away from the problem for a while and think about it from different points of view and about the advantages and disadvantages of possible solutions.

A good listener should make a conscientious effort to evaluate the logic, feelings and credibility of what is heard. The mind functions at some 500 words per minute, but people normally speak at 125 words per minute. In other words, people can think four times faster than they can speak. Rather than letting their minds become bored, people can take advantage of this time differential between thinking and speaking. This time can be used to attempt to anticipate the speaker's next point, attempt to identify supporting materials and mentally summarize what the speaker has said.

LISTENING RESPONSES

One of the deceptive features of listening behavior stems from the speaker's comparative lack of feedback. Feedback enables one to make sure that the message transmitted

---

Feedback enables one to make sure that the message transmitted was received the way it was intended to be received.

---

was received the way it was intended to be received. Feedback via a listening response is a brief comment or action made to another person to convey the idea that the recipient is interested and attentive and wants the

person to continue. The response is made quietly and briefly, so as not to interfere with the speaker's train of thought. It is usually made when the speaker pauses.

The following are the five types of listening responses:

1. nod—nodding the head slightly and waiting.
2. pause—looking at the speaker expectantly.
3. casual remark—"I see," "Uh-huh," "Is that right?"
4. query—asking genuine questions.
5. paraphrasing—repeating back to the speaker your understanding of what has been said.

Each communicative act can involve at least six interpretations (Figure 1).

A simple exercise can be used to demonstrate that often a conscious effort is needed to avoid misinterpretation. When a supervisor is listening to an employee in a discussion, debate or argument, before replying to the employee's comments, the supervisor should repeat what the employee has said. In turn, before the em-

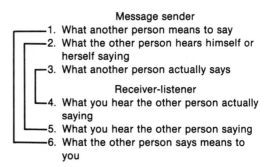

Message sender
1. What another person means to say
2. What the other person hears himself or herself saying
3. What another person actually says

Receiver-listener
4. What you hear the other person actually saying
5. What you hear the other person saying
6. What the other person says means to you

Figure 1. Interpretation of a communicative act.

ployee responds to the supervisor, he or she should repeat what the supervisor has said. This process will be both an eye and ear opener.[12]

Finally, people tend to do a thing well when they hold positive views or "labels" about their ability to do it. One cannot do it until one thinks one can. One can only do what one *wills* to do. People who think they are good listeners probably are, and because of this positive label, they make a conscientious effort to listen and live up to their label. If people say they are poor listeners, they have turned off their listening mechanisms.

At a recent health care workshop, after taking a tape-recorded listening test, a nurse remarked, "If I hadn't done well on that test, I would have been very disappointed because I consider myself to be an excellent listener." In other words, she scored as an excellent listener, and her positive attitude toward listening played a key role in her listening effectiveness.

IMPROVING LISTENING HABITS

Most people talk too much. At times judicious silence should be used. Silence is a great way to motivate other people to speak up and to reveal what is on their minds. Most people frame questions to get the answers they want to hear. Questions should be framed to leave the way open for whatever type of answer the other person wants to give. The other person should be allowed the time to finish the answer.

Most people set up communication in counterproductive atmospheres. If possible, the time and place of a conversation should provide comfort and minimum distraction. If communication is an emotion-laden issue, the place should be private so as to protect the dignity of all parties.

Many people let emotional filters get in the way of understanding. People should be honest about their biases. When one feels strongly about a subject, one should be particularly careful. At such times there is a chance that one will misinterpret, misunderstand and miscommunicate. When emotions boil over, it is a good idea to make a mental note regarding the time and place and people involved. One might be able to track down the source of the feelings and isolate the trigger that sets it off.

Most people listen only for facts. They fail to see the topic from the other person's point of view. One should listen for feelings and pay as much attention to the *way* someone else (or oneself) says something as to what is said. Attention should be paid to *all* meanings.[13]

Birdwhistell noted the following in the Paul Swain Lecture Series at North Carolina State University:

[B]ody language and spoken language are dependent upon each other. . . . However, 55 percent of the social meaning in a conversation is transmitted nonverbally, and in its proper context even silence is communication.[14]

Listening makes the people one is listening to feel special; sometimes it enables them to solve their own problems. Perhaps they are in the process of hearing themselves think aloud on the subject for the first time. At such times they might just want others to listen. If one refrains from injecting oneself into the conversation, one might be able to help them resolve their own internal conflicts.

A professional health care supervisor is, at times, paid to listen. During examinations the physician and nurse do not tell patients how they should feel. The patient sends verbal and nonverbal messages, and the medical personnel receive understanding through listening. Too often supervisors do not let others express their true feelings. When they do, a supervisor may quickly categorize those feelings as good or bad. However, a feeling is just that—a feeling. Few people can help the way they feel, and at times like this they require understanding from others.

Studies at the University of Minnesota, confirmed by studies at Florida and Michigan State Universities, showed that people forget one-third to one-half of what they hear within eight hours.[15] The art of listening is a skill, however, and it can be improved. People listen best when they develop a positive attitude toward listening. The first step is to become aware of the fact that listening is not a passive activity. Also, there is little correlation between intelligence and listening. One must *want* to remember.

REFERENCES

1. Conboy, B. *Working Together: Communication in a Healthy Organization* (Columbus, Oh.: Charles E. Merrill Publishing Co. 1976) p. 73.
2. Nichols, R.G. "Listening is a Ten Part Skill." *Nation's Business* (July 1957) p. 56–60.
3. Rankin, P.T. "Listening Ability" in *Proceedings from the Ohio State Educational Conference, Ninth Annual Session* (Columbus, Oh.: Ohio State University 1929) p. 172–183.
4. Darwin, C. *The Expression of Emotions in Man and Animals* (Chicago: University of Chicago Press 1965).
5. Knapp, M.L. *Nonverbal Communication in Human Interaction* (New York: Holt, Rinehart & Winston 1972) p. 119.
6. Ekman, P., Friesen, W.V. and Ellsworth, P. *Emotion in the Human Face: Guidelines for Research and an Integration of Findings* (Elmford, N.Y.: Pergamon 1962) p. 107.
7. Mehrabian, A., and Weiner, M. "Decoding of Inconsistent Communications." *Journal of Personality and Social Psychology* 6 (May 1967) p. 109–114.
8. Simmel, G. "Sociology of the Senses: Visual Interaction" in Park, R.E. and Burgess, E.W. eds. *Introduction to the Science of Sociology* (Chicago: University of Chicago Press 1921) p. 358.
9. Argyle, M. *The Psychology of Interpersonal Behavior* (Baltimore: Penguin 1967) p. 115–116.
10. Argyle, M. and Dean, J. "Eye Contact, Distance, and Affiliation." *Sociometry* 28 (September 1965) p. 289–304.
11. Myers, G. and Myers, M. *The Dynamics of Human Communication* (New York: McGraw-Hill Book Co. 1973) p. 171
12. Metzger, N. *The Health Care Supervisor's Handbook* (Rockville, Md.: Aspen Systems Corp. 1978) p. 62.
13. Munn, H.E., Jr. and Metzger, N. *Effective Communication in Health Care: A Supervisor's Handbook* (Rockville, Md.: Aspen Systems Corp. 1981) p. 66.
14. Birdwhistell, R. *Paul Swain Lecture Series* (Raleigh, N.C.: North Carolina State University 1974).
15. Kramar, J.H. and Lewis, T.R. "Comparison of Visual and Nonvisual Listening." *Journal of Communication* 1 (May 1951) p. 16.

SUGGESTED READINGS

Barker, L.L. *Listening Behavior* (Englewood Cliffs, N.J.: Prentice-Hall 1971).

Byrne, D.P. *Listening* (New York: Longman 1975).

Dominick, B. *How to Make People Listen to You* (Springfield, Ill.: Charles C. Thomas Pub. 1971).

Duker, S. *Listening Bibliography* (New York: Scarecrow Press 1964).

Kerman, J. *Listen* (New York: Worth Publishing Co. 1976).

Mills, E.P. *Listening Key to Communication* (New York: Petrocelli Charter 1974).

Nichols, R.G. and Stevens, L.A. "If Only Someone Would Listen." *Journal of Communication* 6:1 (1952) p. 8.

Nichols, R.G. and Stevens, L.A. "Listening to People." *Harvard Business Review* 35 (September–October 1957) p. 85–92.

Not by words alone

Harry E. Munn, Jr.
Associate Professor
Department of Speech
  Communication
North Carolina State University
Raleigh, North Carolina

EMPLOYEES MAY choose to stop talking, but they do not cease to communicate. Have you, as a manager, had employees refuse to talk to you or at best say very little although you desperately needed more information? You may not have realized it, but those employees were sending you an assortment of nonverbal messages. To quote Freud, "No mortal can keep a secret. If his lips are silent he chatters with his fingertips; betrayal oozes out of him at every pore."[1]

The health care supervisor must remember that a person cannot *not* communicate. How often have you heard a coworker or employee say, "Seeing is believing"; "Did you see the way he acted when I said . . . ?"; or "I can tell by the look on her face." Remember the song that went, "Why do your lips say no, no, no, when your eyes say yes, yes, yes?" Many times we miss the nonverbal messages that

Health Care Superv, 1983,2(1),1–11
© 1983 Aspen Publishers, Inc.

are sent to indicate: "I don't understand"; "Leave me alone"; "Help me—I'm depressed"; or "I think I understand, but tell me more."

PROCESS OF ABSTRACTION

At times, supervisors appear to be not only the victims of their own communicative behavior, but also the victimizers insofar as their behavior negatively affects others. The type of behavior described can create internal and external conflicts that may become irreparable. It is therefore essential to recognize the nonverbal signs of conflict and to correct a situation before serious damage has been done.

This is, of course, easier said than done. People are usually inclined to see only what they want to see and to hear only what they want to hear. We prepare others to see and hear in a certain way, and we allow others to predispose us to see other people as they want us to see them. Our language, abstractions and mental sets (fixed ways of looking at things) cause us to mislead others and also to be misled by them. It takes two to miscommunicate because the source of a message is just as responsible for clear meaning as the receiver.

As communicators, we are constantly abstracting information. We select bits and pieces of verbal and nonverbal information based on our feelings, needs and attitudes toward the sources of that information. Through this selection process, we predispose ourselves to see things in a specific way. Huseman, Lahiff and Hatfield explain this deceptive selection process as follows:

Since one is exposed to thousands of stimuli each day it is not possible to attach meaning to all of them. Thus, selection is inevitable. This determination and selection are made on the basis of which ones are the most meaningful to the receiver.[2]

We see and hear what we want or are prepared to see and hear; we select. No one else does this for us. Consider the triangles shown in Figure 1. Our familiarity with the statements in each of the three triangles predisposes us to read them in a fixed way. Reread them. Do you notice anything unusual? If you noticed the extra word in each triangle, you are more observant than most. People tend to miss the extra word because they are predisposed to see the statements as they would normally see them. This same process takes place

Figure 1.

when interpreting nonverbal messages. We look for the nonverbal message we expect to see, and we sometimes see it whether it is there or not.

Huseman, Lahiff, and Hatfield contend that "an effective communicator is one who remains aware that he is abstracting. The cost of abstracting is that we sacrifice many details, some of which may be relevant to the subject under consideration. This can result in a distorted perception of reality."[3]

Downs states that on the one hand, subordinates will facilitate upward-directed messages that they believe will either please the boss or enhance their own welfare. On the other hand, superiors will suppress messages directed to subordinates if they perceive such messages as having a deleterious effect on themselves or the organization.[4]

This conclusion was supported by Krivonos, who surveyed the findings of upward-communication research and concluded the following:

- Subordinates tend to distort upward-directed information in a manner that pleases their superiors.
- Subordinates tend to tell their superiors what they want them to know.
- Subordinates tend to tell their superiors what they think they want to hear.[5]

These conclusions are not meant to suggest that all employees are dishonest and untruthful. On the contrary, most are direct and honest and can be trusted to provide accurate feedback when it is requested. Yet at times supervisors still receive distorted information. This is because the selection process previously described predisposes supervisors to see what their employees want them to see. Supervisors need to develop an awareness of this phenomenon in order to deal with it.

NONVERBAL FEEDBACK

How then does a health care supervisor cope with the distortion that takes place during the transmission of verbal messages? To cope more ade-

---

To cope more adequately with the distortion that takes place during transmission of verbal messages, the supervisor must develop an awareness that the verbal message is only half the message being sent.

---

quately with this process, the supervisor must develop an awareness that the verbal message is only half the message being sent. The other half is nonverbal. Nonverbal feedback provides supervisors with a tool to discriminate more accurately between what is being communicated verbally and what is being communicated nonverbally. And the supervisor who is able to recognize and respond to nonverbal feedback can anticipate problems and be of more help to employees.

People send messages nonverbally

through facial expression, eye contact, body action, paralanguage (voice inflection), touching and use of space. When verbal and nonverbal messages are congruent, clear, meaningful communication tends to take place. However, when the nonverbal message appears to contradict the verbal message, unclear and faulty communication occurs.

Birdwhistell has noted that:

Spoken language by itself will not give us the full meaning of what the person is saying. Body language alone will not give us total meaning. If we listen to only the words the person is saying, we may get as much distortion as if we only listen to the body language.[6]

IMPACT OF NONVERBAL MESSAGES

Nonverbal behaviors normally have a high degree of credibility for the beholder. Most hospital employee recruiters would probably agree. "I make up my mind fast, in less than five minutes," stated one hospital employee recruiter. "Sometimes I take a second look, but I seldom change my mind." The same sentiment was expressed at a recent workshop of the North Carolina Directors of Personnel Services. One director said, "I look for nonverbal cues to support what is being said. My first impression is based on appearance, facial expression, eye contact and gestures. A sloppy applicant is at a disadvantage, especially at hospitals that don't have dress codes. I believe that clothing is an extension of self

and that nonverbal behavior truly expresses personality and attitude."[7]

This perception, although made by only one personnel director, is not unusual. It is supported by the research of Webster, who found that interviewers formed an initial impression, much of it based on nonverbal behavior, within the first four or five minutes of an interview and then tended to search for additional information that supported their initial impressions.[8]

Mehrabian found that only 7 percent of the impact of the communication was verbal. Another 38 percent was based on paralanguage; the remaining 55 percent was based on facial expression, gestures and body action.[9]

FORMS OF NONVERBAL COMMUNICATION

Facial expression

More than 100 years ago, Darwin wrote *The Expression of Emotions in Man and Animals*, the product of a century-old pursuit and one of the first works on facial expression.[10] Darwin theorized that facial expressions are instinctive and not learned behavior. However, most anthropologists today believe that facial expressions are a result of involuntary reactions in the muscles and nerves of the face and of cultural conditioning governing the expression of emotion.

In American culture, facial expressions play an important role in social communication. Facial expressions can convey true feelings and be useful communicative tools. Unfortunately, however, rules regarding facial expressions seem at times to parallel that of the ancient Greek stoics in that we are taught from childhood to avoid excessively expressive behavior, facial or otherwise. We are taught to show neutrality when we are angry, especially in public places. If we are unhappy, we are urged to show only the slightest sense of sadness in our demeanor. In our culture, as in many others, facial expressions can be masks behind which we hide.

Even with these limitations, however, the face is one of the most reliable of all nonverbal indicators. Knapp noted that the face is rich in communicative potential. It reflects interpersonal attitudes; it provides nonverbal feedback on the comments of others; it is the primary source of information next to human speech.[11]

There are six basic facial expressions: disgust, surprise, happiness, anger, sadness and fear. Several of these expressions can be exhibited at the same time. For example, an individual can simultaneously exhibit surprise and disgust or surprise and happiness.

The problem is compounded when the verbal message seems to conflict with the nonverbal facial expression. If the meaning of the facial expression is clear and the verbal context in which it occurs is not clear, then the face will be the most reliable source.

Ekman, Friesen and Ellsworth conducted an in-depth analysis of all the important studies of facial expression and concluded that "contrary to the impressions conveyed in previous reviews of the literature that the evidence in the field is confusing and contradictory, our reanalysis showed consistent evidence of accurate judgment of emotion from facial behavior."[12] Mehrabian and Weiner found that when exposed to an inconsistent message, facial expression has the greatest impact, vocal expression has the second greatest and verbal expression has the lowest impact.[13]

Eye contact

A look is more than just seeing. Meaning is constantly being conveyed in visual ways, for example, through the stern look of a boss, the loving look of a patient's relative or the cooperative look of a coworker. Eye contact is a highly personalized form of nonverbal communication. It tells us how we are doing and what kind of relationship we have with another person.

Argyle tells us that there is more mutual eye contact between friends than in other relationships, and persons who seek eye contact while speaking are regarded as being more believable and earnest.[14] We tend to look at things that we like or find attractive and look away from things that we dislike or find unattractive.

Research also indicates that our pupils dilate when we see something or someone we like or find attractive.[15]

Adams found that when two people like one another, they establish eye contact more often and for longer periods of time than when there is tension or dislike in the relationship. She also found that pupil constriction was a sign of emotional aversion.[16] Hess and Polt found that both male and female subjects' pupils dilated in response to pinups of the opposite sex. They concluded that pupil dilation was a reliable index of positive emotional arousal and interest.[17]

Over the past decade, the advertising industry has spent vast sums of money in pupillometry (pupil size as it fluctuates after observing different types of stimuli) research to ascertain its usefulness as a diagnostic tool. Kahneman et al. found that pupil size was a more accurate index of arousal than heart rate or blood pressure.[18]

As early as 1921 Simmel reported: "The mutual glance between persons signifies a unique union between them. By the glance which reveals the other, one discloses himself. The eye cannot take unless at the same time it gives."[19]

Could this be why staring too long at someone causes discomfort? We may look for nonverbal messages in facial expression or pupil dilation, but we may not want to look too long for fear that the other person will see too much of us.

Body action

Health care supervisors, like everybody else, are constantly sending messages with their bodies. To a large extent, a person's social identity and self-image are created by body movements. A supervisor's body actions during conversation with an employee may be a cue to the employee that it is his or her turn to talk. Conversely, a supervisor may send an employee cues indicating that he or she would like to comment on what has just been said.

The next time you have a small group meeting note the body actions of the group members. Employees who seem involved in what is being said and done at the meeting have a tendency to lean forward, and their motions tend to depict an involvement in the interactions that are taking place. In other words, the group dynamics are positive. The opposite behaviors are exhibited by bored group members; they tend to lean away from the discussions taking place. Their body actions depict apathy and disinterest in what is being said and done. Nonverbal cues, such as body position and head movement, express the attitudes that we have, both positive and negative, toward someone who attracts attention as soon as he or she walks into a room.

The body action that is most talked about is the crossing of the arms. It is readily interpreted as a sign of defensiveness, but sometimes the speaker is not being defensive at all. He or she may just feel comfortable talking to someone while in that position. When observing and attempting to interpret nonverbal behaviors, it is always unwise to form broad generalizations about the behavior being observed. Rather, the behavior must be considered in light of other interactions that are taking place. The accuracy of our information will increase when we consider all of the data and how they interact.

Paralanguage

Often, it is not what you say that counts but how you say it. Different

---

Often, it is not what you say that counts but how you say it.

---

tones of voice convey different meanings. We use our voices to regulate conversation. We disclose our emotional states through speech volume, timbre, rate, inflection and enunciation. The behavior of the sender as seen or heard by the receiver results in behaviors that are seen as anger, happiness, boredom, interest, love, hate, frustration or uncertainty.

During telephone conversations, we rely heavily on paralanguage, as such conversations do not allow us to see gestures, facial expression or body actions. It is important to note not only what an individual has to say, but how he or she says it. It is important to keep in mind that paralanguage is the second most important indicator of nonverbal meaning.

Touch

Some everyday expressions indicate the importance of touching in daily living: "Keep in touch." "He's a little touched." "That really touched me." "Don't be so touchy." "That was a touching story." Nonverbal communication often creates a kind of intimacy seldom achieved by words alone.

In patient care, for example, touching often becomes an important way of communicating. Although eye contact is highly personalized, touching is the most intimate way of communicating through the senses. For example, Aguilera found that touching by nurses increased verbal output by patients and improved patients' attitudes toward the nurses.[20]

Often a health care supervisor will not just compliment an employee on doing a good job. He or she will accompany the compliment with a handshake, pat on the back or slight squeeze of the arm or shoulder. It is interesting that it is usually the supervisor who assumes the right to initiate any touching.

Touching is potentially the most threatening type of nonverbal behavior because it can degenerate into object-like control of other people. It can lead other persons to feel that they are being manipulated. Conversely, when a supervisor's tactual contacts reflect genuine feelings, the employee feels confidence, acceptance and encouragement—and responds accordingly. So much has been publicized about sexual harassment in the past several years, however, that most supervisors are reluctant to exhibit any nonverbal sign of appreciation for work well done, for fear that it may be misinterpreted.

Use of space

Space cannot only communicate the intimacy of a relationship, it can also communicate status. One of the earliest mentions of space as a communicative variable is in the Gospel of Luke (14:1–11):

When thou are invited to a wedding feast, do not recline in the first place, lest perhaps one more distinguished than thou have been invited by him. And he who had invited thee and him, come and say to thee, "Make room for this man" and then thou begin with shame to take the last place. But when thou art invited, go and recline in the last place; that when he who invited thee comes in, he may say to thee, "Friend go up higher!" Then thou wilt be honored in the presence of all who are at the table with thee. For everyone who exalts himself shall be humbled, and he who humbles himself shall be exalted.

At one time or another, all of us have had bosses who sat and chatted with us on an office couch—until the subject turned to money or promotion. At that point, they usually moved behind their desks to carry on the conversation, while we remained on the couch. In such instances, space can be seen as representing status. All of us carry our personal space and status with us as we stake out the limits of our influence.

Hall believes that the distance people stand or sit from one another indicates how well they know and how well they like one another. Individuals send nonverbal messages by placing themselves in certain spatial relationships with one another.[21]

White conducted an experiment in a physician's office. He found that when a desk separated physician and patient, only 10 percent of the patients were perceived to be at ease. When the desk was removed, the at-ease state of patients rose to 55 percent.[22]

Distance and space are also strong indicators in working relationships. When we like an employee, we stand rather close and may even touch the person. For example, it seems almost impossible to walk down a hospital corridor with someone you like without bumping shoulders. If you do not like someone, however, it is easy to keep a proper distance.

A personnel director at a North Carolina hospital carried out an interesting experiment. On a piece of paper, he listed the people with whom he worked and to whom he felt close. On that same piece of paper, he also wrote the names of people with whom he worked but to whom he did not feel close. Next he placed a chair by the door to his office, another chair in front of his desk, a third chair at the side of his desk and a fourth one next to his own chair behind his desk. When people entered his office, he did not direct them to any specific chair. After they left, he wrote down which seat each had chosen. As might be predicted, those he felt closest to in his working relationships sat closest to him behind his desk.

Fast described a set of experiments conducted by a professor of psychology at the University of California:

Dr. Sommer entered a hospital wearing a white doctors coat. He then systematically invaded the patients' privacy, sitting next to them on benches and entering their wards and day rooms. The patients reacted to Dr. Sommer's physical intrusions by becoming uneasy and restless and finally by removing themselves from the area.[23]

Because personal space is invisible, people tend to flee rather than fight if an intrusion is made. Personal space may be thought of as a plastic bubble that surrounds the individual. When people meet, they position their bodies so as to keep the walls of the bubbles intact. If one person pushes too close to another, the bubbles bounce apart.[24]

According to Hall, there are three major interpersonal distances that govern Americans' interpersonal relationships: (1) an intimate distance from 3 to 20 inches, (2) a social distance from 20 inches to 5 feet and (3) a public distance from 5 to 100 feet.[25]

CULTURAL DIFFERENCES

Nonverbal behaviors of one ethnic group will not necessarily be the same as those of another. Yet when nonverbal feedback is placed in its proper context, misinterpretation and misunderstandings between different cultural groups can be reduced. For example, people choose their spatial bubbles in light of their own values, mores and cultures. When other people invade their personally created private zones, they become uncomfortable, aggressive and sometimes hostile. For most Americans

engaging in conversation, a distance from two to three feet is comfortable. However, in Brazil, Mexico, France and most Arab countries, a comfortable distance for conversation is less than two feet. In conversation, an American is generally moving backward,[26] while a person from one of the other countries is moving forward.

Nonverbal communicative behaviors must be interpreted in their social context. These behaviors are culturally derived and must be understood by those people, such as health care supervisors, who need to communicate with people from a variety of backgrounds.

Birdwhistell reinforces the point that there are no universal words, no sound complexes, that carry the same meaning the world over. So, too, there are no body actions, facial expressions or gestures that provoke identical reactions in all countries.[27]

PHYSICAL ENVIRONMENT

The complexity of the communication process is often underestimated. In addition to verbal and nonverbal

---

The complexity of the communication process is often underestimated. In addition to verbal and nonverbal messages, physical environment plays a role in that process.

---

messages, physical environment plays a role in that process. Maslow and Mintz explored the emotional responses of participants who attended meetings in beautiful versus ugly rooms. The participants in ugly rooms said the room produced monotony, fatigue, irritability and hostility. Subjects in beautiful rooms reported feelings of pleasure, importance and a desire to continue the activity.[28]

Color affects communicative behavior. The most pleasant hues, in descending order, are said to be blue, green, red and yellow. Red is the most arousing hue, followed by orange, yellow, violet, blue and green.[29]

Amos Alonzo Stagg, one of the most successful coaches in college football history, applied this color concept in his coaching. He had his team's dressing room painted light blue. This pleasant hue had a calming effect on his players during halftime. However, he gave last-minute pep talks in a brilliant-colored anteroom, thereby increasing players' excitement.[30]

CORE PROBLEM

As noted, congruency between verbal and nonverbal messages helps to create clear, meaningful communication. However, not all message-sending is this simple. Company publications, for example, often carry conflicting messages. Redfield has observed that such a publication will often state that "people are our greatest asset," while the front cover shows the new $500 million building without an employee in sight.[31]

More could be said about nonverbal behavior. The core problem, however, may be that while we are still struggling to conceptualize the key communication variable, information, we have too little knowledge of alternate ways of interpreting the various code systems available to people. Those who attempt to abstract meaning from a nonverbal message are merely making an educated guess. Used with discretion and taken in its proper context, however, nonverbal communication can be an effective tool to be used in supervisor–employee relationships.

REFERENCES

1. Brooks, W. *Speech Communication*. Dubuque, Iowa: William C. Brown, 1974, p. 176.
2. Huseman, R.C., Lahiff, J.H. and Hatfield, J.D. *Interpersonal Communication in Organizations*. Boston: Holbrook Press, 1976, p. 27.
3. Ibid., 58.
4. Downs, A. *Inside Bureaucracy*. Santa Monica, Calif.: Rand Corp., 1964, pp. 118–23.
5. Krivonos, P. "Distortion of Subordinate to Superior Communication." Paper presented at a meeting of the International Communication Association, Portland, Oreg., 1976.
6. Birdwhistell, R. *Paul Swain Lecture Series*. Raleigh, N.C.: North Carolina State University, 1974.
7. Anonymous. Comments from the audience of the health care workshop "Improving Your Communication Skills." Wrightsville, N.C.: 1982.
8. Fiedler, F., and Chemers, M. *Leadership and*

Effective Management. Glenview, Ill.: Scott, Foresman & Co., 1974, p. 21.

9. Mehrabian, A. "Communication without Words." *Psychology Today* 2 (December 1968): 53.

10. Darwin, C. *The Expression of Emotions in Man and Animals.* Chicago: University of Chicago Press, 1965.

11. Knapp, M.L. *Nonverbal Communication in Human Interaction.* New York: Holt, Rinehart & Winston, 1972, p. 119.

12. Ekman, P., Friesen, W.P., and Ellsworth, P. *Emotion in the Human Face: Guidelines for Research and an Integration of Findings.* Elmford, N.Y.: Pergamon, 1962, p. 107.

13. Mehrabian, A., and Weiner, M. "Decoding of Inconsistent Communications." *Journal of Personality and Social Psychology* 6 (May 1967): 109–14.

14. Argyle, M. *The Psychology of Interpersonal Behavior.* Baltimore: Penguin, 1967, pp. 115–16.

15. Hess, E.H., and Polt, J.M. "Pupil Size as Related to Interest Value of Visual Stimuli." *Science* 132 (March 1960): 349–50.

16. Adams, R. "Interpersonal Attraction." Paper presented at the 7th National Central Service/ Infection Control Team Conference, Hospital Topics, Kissimmee, Fla., 1981.

17. Hess, E.H., and Polt, J.M. "Pupil Size as Related to Interest Value of Visual Stimuli." *Science* 132 (August 1960): 349–50.

18. Kahneman, D., et al. "Pupillary Heart Rate and Skin Resistance Changes during a Mental Task." *Journal of Experimental Psychology* 79 (January 1969): 164–67.

19. Simmel, G. "Sociology of the Senses: Visual Interaction." In *Introduction to the Sciences of Sociology,* edited by R.E. Park and E.W. Burgess. Chicago: University of Chicago Press, 1921, p. 358.

20. Aguilera, D.C. "Relationships between Physical Contact and Verbal Interaction between Nurses and Patients." *Journal of Psychiatric Nursing* 5 (1967): 5–21.

21. Hall, E. *Hidden Dimensions.* Garden City, N.Y.: Doubleday & Co., 1966): 1–6.

22. White, A.G. "The Patient Sits Down: A Clinical Note." *Psychosomatic Medicine* 15 (May/June 1953): 256–57.

23. Fast, J. *Body Language.* New York: Pocket Books, 1961, pp. 45–46.

24. Sommer, R. "Studies in Personal Space." *Sociometry* 22 (June 1959): 247–60.

25. Hall, E. *Silent Language.* New York: Fawcett Premier Books, 1959, pp. 163–64.

26. Ibid.

27. Birdwhistell, R. "Background to Kinesics." *Etc: A Review of General Semantics* 13 (February 1955): 10–18.

28. Mintz, N.L. "Effects of Esthetic Surroundings: II. Prolonged and Repeated Experience in a Beautiful and Ugly Room." *Journal of Psychology* 41 (April 1956): 459–66.

29. Ibid.

30. Ketcham, H. *Color Planning for Business and Industry.* New York: Harper & Brothers, 1958, p. 114.

31. Redfield, C. *Communication in Management.* Chicago: University of Chicago Press, 1958, pp. 141–42.

Interviewing skills: selecting the right candidate

Norman Metzger
Vice-President for Labor Relations
The Mount Sinai Medical Center
Professor
Department of Health Care
Management
The Mount Sinai School of
Medicine
New York, New York

HEALTH CARE supervisors assume responsibility for employees who are already in place, and their only chance to select *their own* employees is when turnover produces job openings. A supervisor's first opportunity to affect the mix of employees—to build an effective work team—is in the process of selection. The final responsibility for choosing new employees lies with the immediate supervisor, and the employment interview is one of the most important responsibilities of supervision today. Interviewing without thoughtful preparation is a dangerous game. It therefore behooves all supervisors to become acquainted with the tools for improving the effectiveness of selection.

This article was adapted from a chapter in the second edition of The Health Care Supervisor's Handbook *by Norman Metzger and Published by Aspen Publishers, Inc.*

Health Care Superv, 1982;1(1):41–50
© 1982 Aspen Publishers, Inc.

PREPARING FOR THE INTERVIEW

The purpose of the placement interview is to determine specifically, and in as much depth as possible, whether the applicant's work habits, attitudes and personality are compatible with the job to be filled. The supervisor who wishes to be effective in the employment interview should first set a plan for the interview and review in advance the approach to be taken to obtain maximum information and cover all necessary areas. Next the job specifications or job description should be reviewed. This is a critical step; nothing will detract more from positive results in interviewing than to enter the employment interview with only superficial knowledge of the job requirements. If the personnel department has not provided job descriptions, then the supervisor should write them. The application should be reviewed before the arrival of the applicant. If there were any tests administered by the personnel department or any reference checks made in advance, these should be reviewed as well.

The interview should be conducted in an appropriate place. It should be held in private, and phone calls should be limited. The latter are very disturbing to the applicant as well as to the interviewer's train of thought. Adequate time should be alloted for the interview; an average interview should take from 30 to 45 minutes.

The interviewer should be familiar with the five logical segments of the employment interview: (1) warm-up stage; (2) applicant-talking stage; (3) questioning stage; (4) employer-informational stage; and (5) wind-up stage. The interviewer should take care to control the level of his or her language. It is important to speak *to the applicant*, not over or below his or her level.

The interviewer should be careful not to let personal biases get in the way of the selection of the most eligible and most qualified applicant. Finally, the interviewer should not be hesitant about making notes. A record of essential facts and judgments should be made during and after the interview.

CONDUCTING THE INTERVIEW

An interview has four major purposes: to get information, to evaluate

---

An interview has four major purposes: to get information, to evaluate the applicant, to give information and to make a friend.

---

the applicant, to give information and to make a friend. The problem with many interviews is that one or two of these major purposes may be satisfied while the rest remain uncovered. A supervisor who wants to make an intelligent placement judgment must obtain maximum information from the applicant. This will require acute and sensitive listening habits.

Listening

Ralph Nichols, professor of speech at the University of Minnesota, several years ago suggested that people analyze their listening habits with this checklist:

1. Science says that you think four times faster than another person ordinarily talks to you. Do you use this excess time to turn your thoughts elsewhere while you are keeping track of the conversation? (Not a good idea.)
2. Do you listen primarily for facts, rather than ideas, when someone is speaking? (You can miss the essence of the presentation if you do that.)
3. Do certain words, phrases, or ideas so prejudice you against a speaker that you cannot listen objectively to what is being said? (Listen for *what* is said, not for *how* it is being said.)
4. When you are puzzled or annoyed by what someone says, do you try to get the question straightened out immediately—either in your own mind or by interrupting the speaker? (Not a good idea. Wait until the speaker finishes to clarify what has been presented.)
5. If you feel it would take too much time and effort to understand something, do you go out of your way to avoid hearing about it? (Invest the time, and face up to even uninteresting or time-consuming communication.)

6. Do you deliberately turn your thoughts to other subjects when you believe a speaker will have nothing particularly interesting to say? (You may be surprised! Do not judge by first impressions.)
7. Can you tell by a person's appearance and delivery that he or she won't have anything worthwhile to say? (Don't let your biases get in the way of listening.)
8. When someone is talking to you, do you try to make him or her think that you are paying attention when you are not? (It's your loss in the final analysis.)
9. When you are listening to someone, are you easily distracted by outside sights and sounds? (Good listening habits require discipline.)
10. If you want to remember what someone is saying, do you think it's a good idea to write it down as you hear it? (Although notes may be indicated, be careful about paying too much attention to what you are writing and not to what is being said.)[1]

The ratio of interviewer talking to interviewer listening is critical. For the average 45-minute interview, a satisfactory procedure would keep the applicant talking for more than half the time.

Michaels suggests that the interview should actually be an analysis designed to determine the candidate's chances for success. He offers seven primary criteria in the form of questions to be used to draw the critical information from the applicant and enable the interviewer to make a sound hiring decision.

1. Has the applicant performed in a similar capacity?
2. How does the applicant feel about his or her present job?
3. Why does the applicant desire a change in jobs at this time?
4. Do you find the applicant likable?
5. What are the applicant's career objectives?
6. Will the applicant maintain good relations with other managers?
7. What is the applicant's level of self-esteem?[2]

Evaluation of the applicant

It is important for the applicant to evaluate the supervisor and decide whether the institution is the one in which to further his or her career aspirations. Therefore it is essential that the interviewee receive basic information about the job, the institution and opportunities for the future. As important as listening to information and giving information is the evaluation process. Too often the interviewer stumbles into the various pitfalls of interviewing that produce an ineffective evaluation of the candidate and poor results from the interview. It is not uncommon for personal bias to intrude on the effective evaluation of a candidate.

Biases can be favorable or un-favorable. An interviewer may *like* certain things about people and therefore be impressed when an applicant produces one of these favorable traits. Such a trait often produces a "halo effect," and all other attributes are not carefully evaluated. Such biases are not always the common and illegal ones, such as racial, religious and ethnic prejudices. Some supervisors are impressed by the way applicants dress. Others are impressed by the way people comb their hair. Still others seem to be extremely affected by speech mannerisms.

There is a counterproductive mythology surrounding stereotypes. There are still interviewers who believe that they can detect the "criminal" type. The dependence on observational clues to determine successful applicants may well have its place in certain jobs, but too many interviewers still harbor prejudice against fat people (they are jovial, or they are lethargic) or against redheads (they are always hotheaded). The *natural* foundations of character judgments are as unreliable as the myths about such judgments. Appearance often cannot be considered a reliable guide to personality traits. The intrusion of personal biases and pseudoscience has produced an alarming proportion of instant decisions.

Very often interviewers allow their initial impressions to influence their final decisions. One researcher found that most personnel interviewers made their decision after just 4 minutes of a 15-minute interview.[3] This tendency is disturbing, since initial impressions are positively or negatively affected by exploration with the candidate over a much longer period. One might be reminded of the silent screen star whose good looks and swashbuckling manner produced an aura of masculinity, as defined in terms of earlier days, but his voice was revealed to be soprano when talking movies were introduced. The opposite is often true as well; an individual who may not look the part may well be the one who succeeds.

Many people believe that the ideal candidate for a specific position is one who has successfully held a similar position in another institution. However, no two institutions are exactly alike, and candidates who may have had difficulty in one institution could blossom in another. Josefowitz has identified a phenomenon that she calls *the clonal effect*. People tend to hire in their own image. Groups and organizations are inclined to replace lost members with persons having similar characteristics or to add people who will not appreciably change the existing pattern of communications. Cloning tends to reduce diversity and therefore may have an impact on the extent of creativity in an organization. Josefowitz warns that the clonal effect originates mostly in the unconscious. She suggests that supervisors should consciously and actively look for the discomfort of diversity, the challenge of the different and the potential for disagreement.[4]

Public relations

Supervisors should keep in mind that an applicant, even though not successful, is often a member of the community served by the institution. Impressions gained in interviewing for positions are lasting ones. For the individual who is not hired, common courtesy, a dignified approach and a sympathetic rejection will be long remembered even though the job was not offered. For the applicant who is successful, first impressions of the institution—usually obtained in an initial interview—are brought into the work area and can be positive or negative influences in the development of the employee. When interviewing an applicant for employment, the supervisor is both a supervisor of a specific functional area and a public relations arm of the institution. A dignified interview with ample opportunity for the applicant to present his or her credentials will provide immeasurable encouragement to the new employee.

THE USE OF THE APPLICATION FORM

The personnel department is responsible for attracting as many qualified applicants as possible. Selection, which is the supervisor's responsibility, lets only the qualified applicant through the sieve. It is in this selection process that the supervisor attempts to appraise qualities the institution feels are indicative of success on the job. It is critical that the supervisor define in advance what those qualities are. The entire selection process necessitates the making of a value judgment, a forecast as to which applicants will turn out to be productive employees. Mandell states:

[T]he application form plays a simple and important role in selection. Its contents can discourage unsuitable applicants and its design can reflect the company's dignity, reduce to a minimum the time needed to fill it out, and simplify its review. Its wording and its comprehensiveness affect the efficiency and validity of the selection process.[5]

It is imperative that supervisors analyze their institutions' application forms and make constructive suggestions as to design. If the application form is properly designed, it will greatly reduce the time required for the interview. Does the application provide definitive indicators that the supervisor can quickly interpret? The primary objective of the application blank is to compare the applicant's qualifications with the qualifications required for the available job. The application form is the primary written record for preparing the supervisor for the interview.

Pell offers some advice about the use of the application.

1. Use the application form to provide you with the necessary information to evaluate an applicant.
2. Use it as a *guide* to the interview.
3. Read the application form be-fore you start the interview; review it carefully and compare substantive material with job specifications.
4. From the application form, evaluate the applicant's progress in his or her career in relation to education, earnings and work experience.
5. Remember that the résumé or application is written to present the applicant's background favorably. Read between the lines. Keep in mind that what the applicant presents to you on paper is important, but what he or she has omitted is equally important.
6. Do not assume an applicant is a job-hopper solely on the basis of work record; check the reasons for job changes.
7. Do not be overly impressed by superficial aspects of the résumé or application.
8. Do not eliminate an applicant solely on the basis of the application; the interview will tell you a great deal more than the application.[6]

THE FIVE STAGES OF THE INTERVIEW

The interview has been described as a conversation with a purpose. There are four objectives of the selection interview. The first is to match people with jobs. The second is to create good feeling toward the institution. The third objective is to dispense job and institutional information to provide the applicant with a factual basis for accepting or rejecting employment, if offered. The fourth is to provide the interviewer with an opportunity for obtaining data useful for making sound employment decisions, such data not being available from other sources.

The interview logically breaks down into five separate but somewhat overlapping phases: (1) the warm-up stage; (2) the getting-the-applicant-to-talk stage; (3) the drawing-out stage; (4) the information stage; and (5) the forming-an-opinion stage.

Warm-up stage

Most applicants are tense, and unless such tension is relieved, the quality of the interview will suffer. The obvious need to discuss personal information in an interview mandates complete privacy. It is important that the interview be held in uninterrupted privacy to develop a closer relationship with the interviewee. Informality is an important adjunct to this getting-acquainted stage. Talk can be about the weather or about how the applicant traveled to the institution for the interview. Small talk is not inappropriate.

The interviewee is nervous. He or she should not have to sit and wait while the interviewer looks over the application. The interview should not begin with a caustic or insensitive question. The warm-up stage is an investment. The interviewer moves on to the next stage when the applicant is talking and freely exchanging information.

Getting-the-applicant-to-talk stage

The second stage is devoted to starting the applicant talking. This can be done by the use of open-ended questions. It is a good idea to prepare questions in advance of the interview. Care should be taken not to overload the applicant with a series of rapid-fire questions so that he or she is forced to remember the three or four questions posed in succession. Leading questions or questions inviting yes-or-no answers are not the best for this part of the interview. A leading question is often posed to obtain the answer that the interviewer would prefer and is not a good idea. The question with a yes-or-no answer does not have any probing value.

During this part of the interview, the interviewer must be disciplined to balance the amount of intrusion on his or her part. The applicant should dominate this stage of the discussion. The successful interviewer speaks far less than the applicant, even when giving information about the job.

The successful interviewer speaks far less than the applicant, even when giving information about the job.

Drawing-out stage

The third stage is for drawing out the applicant. The interviewer should attempt to elicit answers that were not developed by the applicant when she or he presented background information. Here probing questions are useful. These are incisive and specific questions used to obtain more detailed information on specific activities or topics. When a probing question is asked, the interviewer should be quite familiar with the area being examined. Questions requiring clarification and reflection are also useful at this stage. This type of question essentially "mirrors" the interviewee's answers and is used to get a fuller understanding of the previous answer. It is critical to present the interviewee with a clear indication of genuine interest in his or her background. It is helpful for the interviewer to imagine himself or herself in the applicant's position. The interviewer should not become argumentative in the drawing-out stage. In the event of disagreement, it is not essential that the interviewer correct the applicant or argue. If the interviewer feels that the applicant is holding back information and not telling the complete truth, it may be best to avoid a confrontation and assume a sympathetic posture.

Information stage

In the information stage the interviewer presents a picture of the institution and the specific job under discussion. The interviewer should remember that there are two decisions that must be made in the selection process: (1) whether the applicant should be offered the job and (2) whether the applicant wants to work

in the institution. The interviewer must present the applicant with all pertinent information and answer any questions the applicant may have. This part of the interview can be crucial, since the questions posed by the applicant may reveal a great deal about his or her needs, fears and aspirations. Too often this part of the interview is rushed or underrated; too many times a newly hired employee has said that the job actually performed is quite different from the job explained during the interview.

The job description can be of primary assistance in this stage, since it often contains a summary section and gives the applicant an overall idea of the purpose, nature and extent of the tasks to be performed. Applicants should be absolutely certain about the duties and requirements of the jobs for which they are being interviewed; informing them is the responsibility of the supervisor who will make the placement choice.

Forming-an-opinion stage

The last stage of an interview involves formulating an opinion. Notes can be taken during the interview and used for review in making one's final decision. In reviewing the interview, the interviewer should evaluate the following as evidenced by the answers on the application and the responses during the interview:

- *Previous experience.* Here one should consider whether the applicant had performed similar job duties, had worked under similar working conditions and had the same degree of supervision exercised or received.

- *Education and training.* What were the individual's feelings and reactions concerning her or his educational experiences? These can often give additional information on the attitude that may be brought to the job. Why did the applicant leave school (if she or he in fact did), what subjects did the applicant like best and why, and what subjects did the applicant like least and why? Gaps in educational experience should be explained.
- *Manner and appearance.* What was the impression made by the applicant's general appearance, speech, nervous mannerisms, self-confidence and aggressiveness? Is the applicant's personal appearance suitable for the position? Did the applicant seem nervous and tense throughout the interview? Did the applicant reveal any idiosyncracies?
- *Emotional stability and maturity.* Consider friction with former supervisors, relationships with peers, reasons for leaving jobs and job stability. Consider sense of responsibility and attitudes towards work and family.
- *Supervisory potential.* Consider

previous leadership experience and degree of aggressiveness and self-confidence.

SUCCESSFUL INTERVIEWING

There are a few other considerations that can assist the supervisor in conducting a successful interview. The interview procedure should be neither overly rigid nor too comfortable a routine for the interviewer. The interviewer should avoid excessive formality, since it is essential that the applicant be put at ease. However, the interviewer must maintain control over the course of the interview.

The interviewer should not be impatient. The interview should be as long as necessary to develop a proper evaluation of the candidate. The applicant should be encouraged to speak more than the interviewer. The latter should talk about one-third of the time, certainly less than half the time.

The supervisor should take care not to set the standards for the job too high or too low and should not overhire. Finally, affirmative action is mandated by federal, state and local laws, presidential executive orders and court decisions. Those in a position to hire employees must become knowledgeable about such regulations.

REFERENCES

1. Merrihue, W.V. *Managing by Communication* (New York: McGraw-Hill Book Co. 1960) p. 21–22. (© 1960 by McGraw-Hill Book Co.).

2. Michaels, T.D. "Seven Questions That Will Improve Your Managerial Hiring Decisions." *Personnel Journal* 59 (March 1980) p. 199–200, 224.

(Reprinted with permission of *Personnel Journal,* Costa Mesa, California. All rights reserved.)

3. Webster, E.C. *Decision Making in the Employment Interview* (Montreal: Industrial Relations Center, McGill University 1964) p. 13–14.

4. Josefowitz, N. "The Clonal Effect In Organizations." *Management Review* 68 (September 1979) p. 21–23.

5. Mandell, M.M. *Choosing the Right Man for the Right Job* (New York: American Management Association 1964) p. 158.

6. Pell, A.R. *Recruiting and Selecting Personnel* (New York: Simon & Schuster 1969) p. 101. (© 1969 by Simon & Schuster. Reprint by permission of Monarch Press, a Simon & Schuster division of Gulf & Western Corporation.)

The appraisal interview: Constructive dialogue in action

Jeanne Mancision
Associate Director
Medical Records Services
Columbia-Presbyterian Medical Center
New York, New York

I F WE MAKE THE analogy that the performance appraisal process is similar to the construction of a wheel, we might say that the appraiser is the hub of that wheel. We can have a well-organized, well-documented system, using state-of-the-art forms, scales, and formulas that clearly gather and convey accurate information. However, if the appraiser cannot collect the information and communicate it in an effective manner, the goals of the performance appraisal (PA) may not be achieved. An essential component of a successful appraisal lies in the appraiser's ability to communicate information and to encourage open dialogue.

COMMUNICATING INFORMATION

Dialogue is the key concept. Communication is a two-part process consisting of sending a message and receiving a message. We know how the message has been received by the feedback conveyed by the receiver. We are always communicating. "One cannot *not* communicate. Silence communicates fear, stub-

Health Care Superv, 1991, 10(1), 41–50
©1991 Aspen Publishers, Inc.

bornness, or uncooperativeness. Our choice is not between communicating but between communicating effectively or ineffectively."[1(p.79)] The appraiser must convey, both verbally and nonverbally, a sincere interest in sharing information, and most importantly, in accepting information.

Receiving information often requires patience and tact because speakers can be unclear as to what they are trying to communicate. Listening to what is not being said and observing body language are important ingredients of successful communication. Effective interpersonal skills are a manager's strongest asset, and if these skills emanate from a sincere appreciation of the "human being, warts and all," fruitful communication is assured.

Effective communication is the result of the appraiser's knowledge and understanding of self. Understanding interactions with others is contingent on an increasing awareness of personal feelings and confronting those that obstruct creative vision. Appraisers are not perfect people. They come to each experience with a lifetime of previous experiences that have produced opinions, judgments, and biases. It is important for the appraiser to develop a knowledge and acceptance of these facts in order to conduct an appraisal interview appropriately.

RATING METHODS

The appraiser or rater is generally the immediate supervisor of the employee who is receiving the evaluation. It would seem that the supervisor would be the person who knows the job description and the employee the most thoroughly. It has been shown, however, that "A typical manager has limited contact with his or her employee. Recent studies of how managers actually behave show that managers spend only 5 percent to 10 percent of their workweek with any one subordinate."[2(p.60)] Of course, with different types of management styles, this percentage could increase. For instance, by using Management by Walking Around (MBWA), the manager would hopefully spend more time with the employee. In order to perform an adequate performance appraisal, it is essential that the rater know not just the job description but the individual employee as well. Appraisers must know who and what the person is, in addition to what he or she does, before they can evaluate fairly.

A multiple-rater system can also be used to rate performance. "The idea here is to capture several perspectives on an employee's performance so that a larger number of important performance factors are reviewed and the overall ratings are more accurate."[3(p.66)] While the possibility of having several perspectives may offer a fairer rating, biases can also become more apparent because there is little chance that a rater may be called on to explain an individual decision. In the end, one rater must discuss the appraisal with the employee. This rater may find it difficult to explain and to justify such a group-oriented document.

Peer ratings may have their place in certain settings along with subordinate ratings. However, they are not widely used.[4] Self-rating, as part of the appraisal process, is also helpful. The appraiser gives the appraisee a blank copy of the form to be used in the evaluation. The employee has the opportunity to rate himself or herself and then to discuss the results with the appraiser.

Even though there are various methods of rating, one might wonder whether bias can ever be completely eliminated. And one might also ask whether bias should be completely eliminated. There may be a certain amount of subjectivity that is desirable in such an appraisal, given that we are all ultimately individuals. After all, subjectivity recognizes that "people are not only rational and fallible but are also responsive to real and perceived pressures in PA."[3(p.61)]

TRAINING

Regardless of the type of rating system utilized, the rater must be clear about the overall objectives. To that end, the rater should participate in an adequate PA training program. A good training program is one that gives "information such as the rationale behind the PA program, the policies and procedures to be followed in conducting PA, and an explanation of the terms used in the PA forms and accompanying materials."[3(p.104)] Appraisal skills, consisting of rating and feedback skills, need to be cultivated and tested. Role playing and interview rehearsals using videotape replay are valuable teaching tools for managers to experience. Hopefully, through practice and repetition, managers will gain some familiarity with the process and problems associated with it. Managers can also learn to identify those particular issues that may be personally difficult to address. It is believed that "initial training in performance appraisal should begin early in a manager's career. Introducing training at this stage allows for two distinct benefits. First, the manager becomes aware of the proper performance weights sooner. And second, early training should reduce the likelihood of managers developing bad evaluation habits that are hard to break over time."[5(p.78)] Management commitment is important to the success of the PA program, and dedication to the training needed is an indication of how important management perceives the endeavor. This function should also be recognized as a relevant managerial responsibility, rather than as a troublesome

task required by management and accrediting agencies.

Managers should be trained in the art "diary keeping procedures to increase observational skills."[6(p.205)] In addition, there should be "establishment of a common rater frame of reference to enhance agreement on what constitutes effective job performance."[6(p.205)] Lastly, there should be "mastery based training to increase raters' self-efficacy regarding negative appraisal

---

Negative attitudes toward the performance appraisal program can be altered through training.

---

situations."[6(p.205)] Negative attitudes toward the performance appraisal program can be altered through training. Nevertheless, we realize that we will probably always regard performance appraisal as a necessary, yet tedious, task that "comes with the territory." Mintzberg's study found that "the manager's job most often consists of brief, varied and fragmented activities and that managers prefer current issues and nonroutine tasks.... Traditional PA is a formal organizational procedure, it is highly structured and at least an annual routine."[3(p.99)] The importance of the performance appraisal and its relevance to organizational goals need to be emphasized so that managers stop seeing this function as the emotional and frustrating task that it can be if it is not handled properly. Yearly refresher courses should also be offered on the PA process.

FEEDBACK

The goals of performance evaluation include ensuring that "employees know what they are supposed to do, how well they are supposed to do it, and how they must conduct themselves, assessing performance, recognizing employee accomplishments, determining training and development needs, and documenting factors to support administrative action, i.e., merit pay."[2(p.115)] These goals are accomplished in varying degrees depending on how well the feedback mechanism is utilized. Feedback is essential in order to increase employee understanding, and it is particularly important in performance appraisal. Feedback should occur consistently throughout the employee's professional life. On the day of the formal performance evaluation, the employee should not receive any surprises; throughout the year, the employee should have clearly understood how the supervisor viewed his or her performance. In addition, feedback should be timely. It should occur as close to the actual event being discussed as possible in order to have the strongest impact. Day-to-day performance feedback, in an informal setting, is a very valuable tool. Getting the most out of the feedback mechanism occurs when the manager is descriptive rather than evaluative, when the feedback is specific and timely, when it considers the receiver's needs, when the appraisee is included in the improvement plan and when the appraiser makes reasonable requests.[1]

It is crucial that the employee understand the feedback. To ensure this, the rater might ask the employee to explain his or her understanding of what was written or spoken. While it is easier to provide feedback when it is positive, negative feedback also needs to be shared. Negative feedback can be relayed in the least painful way by evaluating "skills and abilities, rather than attitudes"[7(p.58)] and by trying not to interpret performance.

Coaching is a means by which feedback can be offered consistently throughout the year. Coaching is an "ongoing face-to-face process

of influencing behavior."[2(p.83)] With this process, the manager interacts frequently with the employee (on a daily basis) and encourages and criticizes as the need arises. It is a supportive technique presumed to help the employee to maximize performance for the good of both the employee and the organization.

COMMON RATER PROBLEMS

The job of the appraiser is a difficult one. Many managers do not like to prepare appraisals. They are afraid they will be unpopular if they provide negative feedback. Some managers are uncomfortable at the prospect of judging others, while others welcome the opportunity to wield power in a punitive way.

Using the rater's position in a counselor mode rather than in a judgmental manner can prove helpful in decreasing rater anxiety. Some raters may give undeserved positive evaluations in order to gain approval and to prevent unpleasant ramifications from upper management. There is also the possibility of rating the employee through the use of "central tendency," which is the "temptation to think of everyone as average."[2(p.56)] Rating employees by their personalities rather than by their performance is also a common error known as the halo effect. When operative, it is common for the rater to "rate the subordinate high or low on all performance measures on the basis of one characteristic."[1(p.65)]

Unrealistic expectation is also a common rater problem. Raters cannot require the employee to perform certain functions if they do not provide the materials, equipment, environment, and so forth. Again, the appraiser needs to remain aware of the importance of controlling the effects of personality and bias. Problems incurred as a result of variance in rating styles can be decreased if the appraiser uses standardized measures for rating performance. Lastly, appraisers should not compare one employee's performance to another's. By recognizing ambiguity throughout the rating process, we take the first step toward eliminating it.

THE PERFORMANCE APPRAISAL INTERVIEW

Both the employee and the appraiser should be prepared for the performance appraisal interview. Guidelines for what the employee and appraiser should do before, during, and after the interview are summarized in Appendixes A and B, respectively. These topics are also discussed in the paragraphs that follow.

Preparing for the appraisal meeting

In preparation for the appraisal meeting, the appraiser has several tasks to complete. First, the employee to be appraised should be notified, in person and in a nonthreatening manner, that a discussion will occur. A mutually convenient date, place, and time should be established for the event, and the employee should be given a blank evaluation form to complete, in addition to a copy of a current relevant job description. The appraiser might also ask the employee to "prepare a list of new objectives for work improvement, new projects, and career development—including a brief outline of plans to specific request for support from you and the other managers."[2(p.117)] Rather than being told that this will be an evaluation, the employee may be asked to regard the purpose of the meeting as a review of last year's work activity, performance, and plans for the future. Including the employee in the preview preparation discourages adversarial and anxious feelings.

The appraiser should also prepare for the event by reviewing the current job description as well as last year's performance appraisal. The rater should be comfortable and familiar with the evaluation form and should review rater training manuals to be reminded of potential rating pitfalls. With adequate preparation, such problems can be avoided. Above all the appraiser should remember that each employee is a distinct individual. Therefore, the review should be tailored to that person. Hopefully, the rater will have accumulated a file of critical incidents that occurred throughout the year, relating to the employee's performance. Attention to material facts rather than irrelevant, subjective conjecture is necessary. Otherwise, the appraiser will appear unprepared and will lack credibility.

The appraiser, after reviewing all information and gathering professional opinions from other managers, if appropriate, rates the employee. Finally, the appraiser reviews the evaluation for completeness and accuracy. In order to be optimally prepared for the interview, the appraiser should "select the exact words for use for introductory statements, to criticize, and to confront defensiveness. Anticipate problems. Be ready to cite specific examples to illustrate your points."[2(p.117)]

Conducting the appraisal meeting

The meeting should take place in a private area without interruptions. The rater can help to create a comfortable and calm environment by initiating a benign conversation and by sitting next to the employee rather than across a desk. The employee is probably quite anxious at this point, therefore the rater should try to show empathy and to help the employee relax.

The rater might begin the interview by outlining the expectations of the meeting, starting with a review of the employee's self-appraisal.

If the self-appraisal is similar to that completed by the rater, there is less chance of a confrontation. The two parties can discuss the differences and work toward a mutual understanding. It is important for the rater to keep the lines of communication open.

Next, the rater presents the evaluation to the employee. The rater should encourage the employee to take ample time to read and to understand the comments. If performance has been acceptable, the rater should compliment the employee. However, the rater should not offer empty compliments in an attempt to buffer negative feedback. The rater should also avoid sandwiching compliments between criticisms. It is important that the rater present an accurate and fair assessment in a supportive and nonpunitive manner.

After both appraisals have been shared and discussed, the appraiser allows the employee to verbally react to the appraisal. If there is disagreement, it is important for the appraiser to be patient and try to understand what the employee is feeling. In fact, the appraiser should repeat what the employee has said so there will be clarity of understanding. When both parties understand one another, it is possible to discuss and to resolve differences.

Negative feedback can provide opportunities for improvement, and conveying this is an art that a sensitive rater must learn to practice. Perhaps the appraiser might want to ask the employee if there are any changes that might enhance job satisfaction and career development. Finally, the appraiser should summarize the meeting, clarify the salient points, and make arrangements for follow-up actions such as additional conferences. If the rater has been able to inspire and motivate the employee and to improve their relationship, the meeting has been successful. It might be helpful for the appraiser to utilize a postinterview checklist in

order to grade his or her own performance.

Often salary and merit increases are discussed at the appraisal interview. Money issues can emit mixed signals to the employee because the financial reward might not be appropriate to the evaluation. Ideally, the appraisal should be conducted separately from the financial discussion, although in some organizations this is not possible. Appraisers can feel frustrated if they do not have the financial means to reward exemplary appraisals. Also, marginal performers may receive substantial increases simply because the organization had a good year. If they must be included, salary issues should not be discussed until the end of the interview. According to Umiker,

Salary should not be discussed at performance appraisal interviews. The introduction of a discussion of salary dominates and distorts the interview. Even worse, it promotes an adversarial relationship in that employees argue for lower, not higher, standards of performance. Furthermore, if employees are told that they are being recommended for a merit raise, they are less likely to place credence in any criticism.[2(p.122)]

The most important aspect of the evaluation is the "exchange of views."[1(p.65)] Maintaining this communication is the key to job improvement and to building a strong working relationship between employee and manager. It has been said that

Supervisors who do a good job in communicating their evaluation of an employee's performance will encourage reactions, face up to and resolve differences and reach mutual understanding of the implications of the review. The successful supervisor is able to communicate to employees who perform below standard and is interested enough to commend those whose performance is above standard.[1(p.69)]

Although it is everyone's wish that the appraisal interview will proceed smoothly, there is the possibility that the employee will not agree with the appraisal. The employee who becomes angry and heated should be allowed to talk it out; the appraiser should not try to stop him or her from venting frustration. In many cases, it is wise for the appraiser to say nothing. If the person becomes increasingly rude or abusive, the appraiser may want to end the meeting and reschedule it for the following day.

An employee may also appear to agree with everything the appraiser says, or the employee may say nothing at all. The rater must encourage dialogue. If there is no verbal communication, distrust and resentment may ensue. The employee may readily agree with negative feedback quickly in an effort to deflect attention from the subject. The astute rater will recognize this tactic and control the dialogue. An employee may also use tangents in an effort to avoid uncomfortable discussions. Again, the appraiser should recognize the dynamics and retain control of the interview.

An employee who is criticized may seek justification in comparisons to others in the department. The appraiser should not be drawn into discussions concerning other behaviors and other employees. Most importantly, the rater should not let a persuasive employee force the alteration of an honest opinion rendered in good faith. Raters may want to be prepared for any and all responses in the appraisal meeting; however, this is not realistic. Moreover, each employee reacts differently to appraisals. The impudent personality may prove taxing if the appraiser is intimidated by aggression and cannot set limits. Employees who need attention and recognition may tediously comment on every aspect of the appraisal. An analytical employee may weigh the pros and cons of the appraisal and then decide whether to accept or reject it. Finally, there is the passive and insecure employee who is probably the hardest to reach. This employee may need urging to participate in open dialogue without fear of reprisal.[8] Knowing the employees and being aware of their strengths and weaknesses, coupled with a sincere desire to create job satisfaction, are ways in which the rater can decrease the amount of negative experiences associated with performance appraisal.

• • •

The rater's role in performance appraisal is pivotal. Providing consistent feedback and winning the trust of the employee by honest and open verbal exchange are deciding factors in the overall success of the appraisal program. The manager must be trained to perform evaluations skillfully and with a commitment to the employee and to the organization. In addition, the appraiser must recognize that actively attempting to improve appraisal skills is a key responsibility of a good manager.

REFERENCES

1. Metzger, N. *The Health Care Supervisor's Handbook.* Rockville, Md.: Aspen Publishers, 1988.
2. Umiker, W. *Management Skills for the New Health Care Supervisor.* Rockville, Md.: Aspen Publishers, 1988.
3. Devries, D.L., Morrison, L.M., Shullman, S.L., Gerlach, M.L. *Performance Appraisal on the Line.* New York, N.Y.: Wiley, 1981.
4. Novit, M.S. *Essentials of Personnel Management.* 2d ed. Englewood Cliffs, N.J.: Prentice Hall, 1986.
5. Regel, R., and Hallman, R. "Gauging Performance Objectively." *The Personnel Administrator* 32, no. 6 (1987): 74–78.
6. Bernardin, H.J., and Buckley, M.R. "Strategies in Rater Training." *Academy of Management Review* 6 (1981): 205–12.
7. King, P. *Performance Planning & Appraisal.* New York, N.Y.: McGraw-Hill, 1984.
8. Bizzatta, M. "Improving Your Performance Appraisal." *Management Review* 77 (1988): 205–12.

SUGGESTED READING

Anderson, G.C., and Barnett, J.G. "Characteristics of Effective Appraisal Interviews." *Personnel Review* 16, no. 4 (1987): 18–25.

Bernardin, H.J., and Buckley, R. "Strategies in Rater Training." *Academy of Management Review* 6 (1981): 205–12.

Bizzatta, M. "Improving Your Performance Appraisals." *Management Review* 77 (1988): 40–44.

Coile, R.C., Jr. *The New Hospital.* Rockville, Md.: Aspen Publishers, 1986.

DeFuria, M.C., and Shinshak, D.G. "Performance Evaluations in Service Systems: A Look at the Health Care Industry." *National Productivity Review* 7 (1988): 318–23.

DeMeuse, K. "A Review of the Effects of Non-Verbal Cues on the Performance Appraisal Process." *Journal of Occupational Psychology* 60 (1987): 247–51.

Denton, K. "How to Conduct Effective Appraisal Interviews." *Administrative Management* 48 (1987): 15–17.

Grant, P. "A Better Approach to Performance Reviews." *Management Solutions* 32 (1987): 11–16.

Regel, R., and Hallman, R. "Gauging Performance Effectively." *The Personnel Administrator* 32, no. 6 (1987): 77.

King, P. *Performance Planning & Appraisal.* New York, NY: McGraw-Hill, 1984.

Locker, M. "Appraisal Trends." *Personnel Journal* 67 (1988): 139–40.

Metzger, N. *The Health Care Supervisor's Handbook.* Rockville, Md.: Aspen Publishers, 1988.

McConnell, C.R. *Managing the Health Care Professional.* Rockville, Md.: Aspen Publishers, 1984.

Novit, M.S. *Essentials of Personnel Management.* 2d ed. Englewood Cliffs, NJ: Prentice Hall, 1986.

Simivas, S., and Motowidlo, S.J. "Effects of Rater's Stress on the Dispersion and Favorability of Performance Ratings." *Journal of Applied Psychology* 72 (1987): 247–51.

Umiker, W. *Management Skills for the New Health Care Supervisor.* Rockville, Md.: Aspen Publishers, 1988.

Appendix A
Performance appraisal interview guide for the employee

BEFORE THE INTERVIEW

1. Know your job description.
2. Ask for a copy of the evaluation and perform your own appraisal.
3. Expect that you will be allowed ample time to prepare.
4. Be sure that the manager performing the evaluation is familiar with you and the quality of your work.
5. Be prepared to discuss your performance.
6. Be prepared to accept and to give constructive criticism professionally.
7. Come to the meeting with potential solutions as well as opportunities for improvement.
8. Think of ways in which management can help you to improve your performance and to decrease frustration.

DURING THE INTERVIEW

1. Engage in benign conversation with the rater.
2. Listen to the agenda for the meeting.
3. Share and discuss your self-appraisal with the appraiser.
4. Listen to the rater's comments.
5. Work with the appraiser toward mutual understanding and an honest and open dialogue.
6. Share your feelings.
7. Offer suggestions.
8. Follow up on your commitment to improved performance.
9. Ask for feedback at regular intervals.

AFTER THE INTERVIEW

1. Expect coaching.
2. Request feedback if it is not consistently offered.
3. Continue to work with the rater toward better communication and mutual understanding.
4. Strive to reach your potential.
5. Explore career opportunities.

Appendix B
Performance appraisal interview guide
for the appraiser

BEFORE THE INTERVIEW

1. Know the employee and the job description.
2. Give the employee notice that the appraisal will occur.
3. Schedule the appointment at a mutually convenient time.
4. Give the employee ample time to prepare.
5. Gather information pertaining to the employee's performance.
6. Refer to the rater training manuals for guidance in avoiding rater pitfalls.
7. Choose a private place.
8. Anticipate reactions, plan the course of the meeting, and try to prepare for any eventuality.
9. Know the company policy regarding salary, merit pay, and appraisal.
10. Give the employee a self-appraisal form.

DURING THE INTERVIEW

1. Do not allow interruptions.
2. Do not rush the interview.
3. Listen to the employee's self-appraisal.
4. Create a comfortable atmosphere.
5. Give the employee his or her evaluation.
6. Invite discussion.
7. Allow time for both parties to discuss views.
8. Be calm, patient, and professional in the face of adversity.
9. Encourage a 50/50 dialogue.
10. Summarize discussion.
11. Make an appointment for follow-up conference.
12. Ask for input regarding your role in job enhancement.

AFTER THE INTERVIEW

1. Critique your performance.
2. Follow up on plans made for future meetings.
3. Provide feedback all year round.
4. Continue to work toward improving relations with the employee.

A giant step toward improved supervisory effectiveness

Charles R. McConnell
Vice President for Employee Affairs
The Genesee Hospital
Rochester, New York

RUNNING ON HABIT

This brief discussion is about one aspect of managerial behavior, represented by a seemingly small pattern of actions that can be summarized in one short sentence. A supervisor who is not operating according to this simple pattern of actions can make a quantum leap toward managerial effectiveness through one modest change in behavior.

Consider the flaws in the following scenarios:

- "Harry," says the distribution manager, "the clutter in the stock room is starting to get away from us, and we need to do something about it. When you get the chance, I'd like you to put together some recommendations for some new shelves and bins and come up with a suggested layout that makes better use of the space we've got."
- "Here, Janet," says Janet's supervisor while handing over several smudged,

Health Care Superv, 1990, 8(4), 71–76
© 1990 Aspen Publishers, Inc.

dog-eared sheets of paper, "as soon as you can, I'd like you to bring our master suppliers list up to date and make certain that all the price lists are current."

- "Bill," instructs the department manager, "we're rolling headlong into budget time again, and I need you to pull together a first draft of our department's nonsalary budget. Any time by the end of this week will be fine." However, Bill is in no great hurry to get started on the budget numbers because he knows through considerable experience that it will be ten to 14 days past "the end of this week" before the manager mentions this particular need again.

What flaws are apparent in the foregoing scenarios? Well, perhaps there will appear to have been no flaws at all. The employees might all respond in a fashion timely enough to meet the bosses' requirements; but then one or more might not.

In each instance the manager is probably acting out of habit, behaving at work essentially the same way he or she would behave at home. In each instance the manager is probably also acting as he or she expects managers to act; that is, deciding what is to be done and giving people orders or instructions. But as common, ordinary, and everyday as these opening scenarios sound, they are flawed in that specific deadlines for action are lacking and there are no indications that the manager will follow up.

IN THE MIND OF THE LISTENER

What is truly meant by "when you get the chance" or "as soon as you can"? These phrases will have different meanings for different people. To some employees, "as soon as you can" means right this minute, to others it means today or tomorrow, and to still others it means days or even weeks. To some employees, "when you get the chance" means tomorrow, next week, next month, or never. In the absence of specific deadlines, employees are left to respond according to how they personally interpret the managers' statements.

Of course, this is saying nothing new about the questionable ways in which much business communication takes place or about the less-than-specific language that is commonplace in our daily work. Just as "when you get the chance" can mean a variety of things to different people, so too do words such as prompt, adequate, sufficient, and appropriate have different meanings or bring to mind different concepts. The true meaning of "when you get the chance" or "as soon as you can" is the meaning of the moment; it is the meaning given those words in exactly that context at exactly that moment by the person who is hearing them.

CONDITIONED EMPLOYEES AND EXPECTATIONS

And what of the specific assignment to be completed by "the end of this week" that the manager does not mention again until another two weeks have passed? Employees tend to respond to a manager according to their expectations of that manager, and if laxity in following up on deadlines is the general practice, they will respond accordingly and use much of the extra time they know is available to them. Of course not all employees will behave in this manner; some will consistently do what they are asked to do on time. However, in the absence of specific deadlines and active follow-up, a considerable number of employees will respond to the manager's laxity with a looseness of their own because they have been conditioned to do so by the supervisor, their most visible role model.

The supervisor and employee in this scenario have become locked into a self-perpetuating cycle in which inappropriate behavior is repeated and repeatedly reinforced: The supervisor mentions a vague deadline or none at all, there is no follow-up, the employee runs late but the supervisor's

---

To some employees, "as soon as you can" means right this minute, to others it means today or tomorrow, and to still others it means days or even weeks.

---

behavior implies that this is acceptable, and so on. Under such circumstances, most employees eventually learn how much time they actually have to do the work that must be done, and what kinds of work need never be done. Many employees eventually settle into doing less than the best they are capable of simply because the supervisor's behavior does not encourage them to produce results within a reasonable time.

THE GIANT STEP: DEADLINES AND FOLLOW-UP

Thus the potential giant step toward improved managerial effectiveness is: For every task that is assigned, set a reasonable deadline; if results are not forthcoming when the deadline arrives, immediately follow up with the employee.

The advice is certainly simple—perhaps simple to the point of seeming unworthy of mention. However, this important bit of behavior is not practiced by a great many managers. What manager has not occasionally directed that something be done "when you get the chance," "when you have a moment," or "sometime soon"? Yet in the absence of a specific deadline, the employee to whom the task is assigned receives a mixed message. Often enough to be chronically troublesome, the message that rises to the surface is: This task is not particularly important.

It is clearly to the supervisor's advantage to behave as though any task that is important enough to be assigned to someone deserves a deadline. For even the most insignificant task, always assign a deadline—even if that deadline is extremely loose. In any case, make the deadline as reasonable for the employee as possible.

Again consider Harry and the stock-room problem of the opening scenario. Today is Thursday, October 8, and the manager has just learned that he must present a stock-room modernization plan at a management meeting on Friday, October 16. He knows that he will have to do some additional work with Harry's input when he has it in hand, so the manager might be inclined to put the pressure on Harry to respond within one or two working days to leave himself some extra time for his own efforts. The manager's deadline of Friday the 16th might then be more than reasonable, but Harry's deadline may be extremely tight.

The manager should split the difference with Harry, according to how much work each has to do, and perhaps call for Harry's input by Tuesday afternoon or Wednesday morning. This would give Harry a reasonable amount of time to do his job but retain enough slack for refinements and contingencies.

There will of course be times when the employee's immediate response is required by factors beyond the manager's control. But otherwise, the manager should not horde the slack but should rather split the available time with the employee to ensure that the deadline is reasonable.

EASY TO SAY, NOT AS EASY TO DO

As any task that is worth assigning is worth assigning a deadline, so too is any assigned deadline deserving of faithful follow-up. The assignment part of this suggestion is the easy part; having decided to do so, to hand out a few specific assignments complete with specific deadlines is simple. However, good intentions break down as old habits reassert themselves, and somehow the follow-up phase of the activity never gets the amount of attention given to the assignment phase.

Faithful follow-up is of critical importance in a supervisor's pattern of behavior; often the failure to follow up on a specific deadline creates a condition that is worse than if no deadline had been assigned at all. Employees readily adapt to a manager's style, so they come to expect that follow-up will be late or nonexistent if that has usually been the case. The resulting procrastination can take such a firm hold on a department that employees do not think about taking extra time—they simply *know*, without conscious thought, that they have more time than the manager's spoken words suggest.

The key word to use in describing this kind of undesirable management behavior is *habit*. A great deal of what most supervisors do is governed by habit, and it is no more than habit that causes a supervisor to deal in vague or nonexistent deadlines and to follow up either late or not at all. To adopt an improved pattern of actions requires the establishment of a new, good habit—or more appropriately, the replacement of some old habits with some new and better ones. This is accomplished by first deciding on a new pattern of actions, and second, reinforcing the new pattern through constant reminders.

Much like the common-sense principles so often espoused for the improved management of time, advice about improving one's use of deadlines and follow-up is easy to dispense and understand but difficult to follow. This difficulty exists because of the extent to which we invariably underestimate the power of habit. The steps required to improve one's use of deadlines and follow-up are simple and few, but their implementation can lead to numerous false starts as we rediscover that a considerable amount of determination and tenacity is required to change a habit.

The only mechanical aid required is a calendar book, preferably one that provides a single page for each day. When an assignment is given to an employee, determine a deadline for completion and enter that deadline on the appropriate page in the calendar book. Do not wait until later to enter the deadline; do not save up a few days' worth of assignments—or even a single day's worth of assignments—with the intention of entering them all at the same time. Rather, as the final step in handing out the assignment enter the deadline on the appropriate day's calendar page. After just a few days of such activity, you may find that your calendar is dotted with deadlines falling due within days, weeks, or even months. Even an assignment of the "nonessential, but nice if we did it" kind, an item of genuinely minimal priority, is deserving of a deadline, even if that deadline is months in the future.

Each day, perhaps at one specific time of day, scan the day's page in the calendar book for those items you assigned as due on that day. If no results have been forthcoming, and if you have not been informed of any unavoidable delays or reasonable readjustment of priorities, faithfully follow up on each deadline.

CHANGING MORE THAN JUST YOURSELF

In implementing this advice in a deliberate, planned effort to improve your effectiveness, begin modestly and give every employee the benefit of the doubt. Timely follow-up might at first be as simple as, for example, Bill's manager seeking him out and saying, "Bill, this is the day we were going to take a look at your first draft of the nonsalary budget. Where does this stand?" Such follow-up, faithfully pursued on a preestablished deadline date, will be sufficient to give most employees the message you want to convey. And certainly after two, three, or four such follow-ups, the majority of employees will get the message and begin responding when they were told to respond.

In changing the way you assign work and following up on those assignments, you are forcing your employees to change the way they respond to you.

It is important to remember that you are changing not just yourself, but all employees who report to you. In changing the way you assign work and following up on those assignments, you are forcing your employees to change the way they respond to you. Under the best of circumstances, many employees are naturally resistant to change; you can expect even greater resistance, or resentment, when change is forced on the employees. Therefore, you need to be flexible. You need to go slowly and provide your employees with plenty of opportunity to recognize what you require of them, and plenty of opportunity to work through their resistance without being penalized for it. In other words, maintain a steady pressure of reasonable assignments and reasonable deadlines, but do not extend criticism for missed deadlines until your habits have permanently changed and your employees are automatically compliant.

PATIENCE AND FAITHFUL FOLLOW-UP

In attempting to change your ways and change the way your employees respond to you, you may be called on to demonstrate a considerable amount of patience. If your past behavior concerning deadlines and follow-up was at all lax, your employees' loose or casual responsiveness is more your fault than it is theirs. In addition to altering a habit of your own, you are making it necessary for employees to alter the way in which they respond to you.

In summary, it bears repeating that any task worth assigning at all is worth giving a reasonable deadline. And having assigned a deadline, never let the deadline pass without following up. Faithfully follow up on every deadline you assign, and you will find that eventually the need for you to follow up on unfulfilled deadlines will all but disappear. Once you have thoroughly incorporated the practice of assigning deadlines and following up on them, you will have taken a giant step toward improved supervisory effectiveness.

Part IV
Of Problems and Groups

Strategies for resolving conflict

Linda G. Bertinasco
Major
United States Air Force Clinic McChord
McChord Air Force Base
Tacoma, Washington

THE EVIDENCE of conflict within hospitals is becoming increasingly apparent. Nurse and nonprofessional hospital employee strikes receive widespread publicity. Conflicts between administrators and medical staff are coming into public view via the media. Hospital-client conflicts are increasing as consumers of hospital services level charges of inefficiency and inattention to consumer expectations. Internally, managers at all levels are faced with eruptions of interpersonal and departmental conflicts.

The demands placed on hospital middle managers have never been greater.[1] The decrease of inpatient census has forced managers to work with diminished resources. Hospital administrators are demanding more accountability and pressur-

The opinions and assertions contained herein are the private views of the author and are not construed as official or reflecting the views of the Department of the Air Force or Department of Defense.

Health Care Superv, 1990, 8(4), 35–39
© 1990 Aspen Publishers, Inc.

ing middle managers to think in terms of cost–benefit ratios, cost accounting, and marketing strategies. Reviews and audits by external agencies have become more frequent and more exacting. How does the hospital middle manager deal with these stressful conditions and the conflicts that arise within the organization? The first step in resolving conflict is to identify the underlying causative forces.

NATURES OF CONFLICT

Hospital-client conflict is allegedly increasing, though few studies have been conducted to examine the problem.[2] Until recently, patients have had little voice in hospital matters, nor did they seem to desire one. The feeling was that professionals knew what was best for patients. The increasing number of malpractice suits may be turning this perception around. A lack of clearly defined community service goals could be an underlying factor in the conflict: Sometimes they become the servants of the organization rather than the master. What is best for an individual hospital might not always be best for the society it serves.

Certain internal characteristics inherent in hospital organizations foster conflict. For example, interdependence, specialization, and various types of personnel and levels of authority all appear to be related to conflict. Hospital size also must be included in this calculation; the larger the facility, the more communication channels must be maintained. Policies and procedures become more formalized with greater hospital size, and less interpersonal contact exists across hierarchical ranks.[3] In fact, few organizations are composed of as many diverse skills as the hospital, which generally has nearly three employees for each patient and a heterogenous health team influenced by more than 300 professional societies and associations.[4]

Interpersonal conflicts in hospitals also seem to be increasing. For this article, the term *interpersonal conflict* includes both interpersonal disagreements over issues and interpersonal antagonisms.

In industry, top executives usually enjoy both formal and informal power and status. This is not true in the hospital organization, where basis of power is derived from legitimacy, control of rewards and sanctions, expertise, personal liking, and coercion. This situation is unique to hospital organizations and is a basic source of administration–medical staff conflict. Recent demands by the American Medical Association and by medical directors in many hospitals call for medical staff representation on hospital boards. This, too, prompts managerial conflict.

As physicians attempt to maintain or increase their power and administrators try to improve their status, both tend to feel threatened.

Professional membership does not necessarily mean harmony among members of a discipline. The ways in which individuals view the roles of others affect conflict. The administrator is a source of influence with authority delegated from trustees, while physicians exercise influence by virtue of their expertise, prestige, status, and power among patients and community. Physicians tend to view administration as a less-prestigious line of work. As physicians attempt to maintain or increase their power and administrators try to improve their status, both tend to feel threatened. Under such circumstances, conflict increases.

Status is a source of basic conflict among nurses.[5] In past years, nursing was one of the few careers a woman could enter in which she could attain some degree of professional prestige. Today, women are gaining increased recognition in fields such as business, government, medicine, and education. Nurses had been virtually the only professionals in the hospital aside from physicians. They are now experiencing increased competition for status from a proliferation of allied health professionals, many of whom enjoy higher standards of education, pay, and autonomy than do nurses. One study showed that, compared with student nurses (who have a relatively high image of nursing on the average), the general-duty nurse has an especially low image of nurses, and other hospital personnel have an even lower image of nursing.[5]

CREATING AN ENVIRONMENT FOR CONFLICT RESOLUTION

There are various strategies for dealing with disruptive situations in organizations. The following will discuss three such strategies: win-lose, lose-lose, and win-win.

The win-lose orientation is demonstrated by autocratic administrative practices in which the administrator feels that any conflict situation is ultimately a personal threat. Staff members who work with a win-lose administrator often develop intense frustrations. They use the strategy of communicating only "what the boss wants to hear," thereby avoiding direct confrontation.

Lose-lose is so named because neither side accomplishes what it wants or, alternatively, each side only gets part of what it wants. Administrators with this orientation assume that "half a loaf is better than none" and prefer avoidance of conflict to personal confrontation on issues.

The primary goal of a win-win strategy is to find high-quality, highly acceptable solutions to organizational problems.[6] To realize this goal, several values need to be integrated into the administrative patterns of the organization.

The first element is related to the administrator's belief that it is possible to find solutions that will be both high quality and highly acceptable. The concept implies that the administrator is willing to look at the goals, motivations, and needs that others bring to the conflict situation. It also implies a realization that the commitment each party feels toward the solution will determine whether a defined solution satisfactorily resolves a given problem.

The second element that must be communicated is related to willingness to foster honest communication. When someone is evasive about the reason a position is strongly advocated, distrust tends to arise. But honesty begets honesty, and when an individual can verbalize feelings, motivations, and perceptions, others in the group generally follow that lead. The result is that the problems can be more sharply defined and the critical issues more openly delineated.

A final necessary element is the conviction that serious problems are best resolved when defined, process-oriented decision-making methods are used. A problem-solving methodology that is defined increases the probability that defensiveness can be diminished and creative solutions can emerge.

If win-win orientations are to become an integral part of administration, three competencies need to be developed and applied to organizational problems: the willingness to adopt and practice a style of confronting, approaching, and managing conflict; the willingness to invest effort in helping others clarify the meaning of messages; and the willingness to follow systematic processes to arrive at high-quality solutions that foster high acceptance.[2]

There are five basic styles of approaching or avoiding conflict-producing situations: withdrawing, smoothing, compromising, forcing, and confronting.

Withdrawal from conflict-producing situations occurs when an administrator will not initiate action unless it is absolutely necessary. When a disturbing memo is received, the answer is deferred or the memo is filed or forgotten. When questions are raised regarding the memo, the individual may reply, "It is being studied" or "I haven't had a chance to read it."

Smoothing occurs when an administrator wishes to avoid disagreement, negative emotions, and frustrations. The emphasis is to accentuate the positive: "Well, I know that we have our problems, but look at all the good things we are doing." This look-at-the-bright-side approach does not necessarily result in a cohesive department, since employees become frustrated when issues are not confronted. Also, it becomes difficult to be angry with the administrator because he or she is perceived as a nice person.

Compromising occurs when an administrator finds a middle position where all parties feel comfortable. The limitation of a compromise approach is the intent to find an equitable solution rather than the best possible solution for the problem. Because the emphasis is on compromise, less effort is expended on the quality of the solution than on how individuals will accept it.

Forcing occurs when the administrator seeks to meet his or her own goals at all costs, without concern for the needs or acceptance of others. Losing is perceived as reduced status; winning brings a sense of achievement. The forcer has no doubt about the correctness of the position, and anger is expressed toward those who disagree.

Conflict is an inherent part of organizational life, and ongoing conflict resolution processes must be developed, implemented, and periodically evaluated. The problem solver who confronts the situation sees conflict as natural and helpful. In this setting, everyone's attitude is aired and everyone shares an equal role in resolving conflict. There are no sacrifices simply for the good of the group. This approach is the most effective in managing conflict resolution.

•   •   •

In thinking through conflict management, there can be no quick fix that is a lasting one. This is not a threat to the integrity of the administrator, but rather a challenge to his or her ability to carry learned principles of management through to a satisfactory conclusion. While communication is only one of the keys to the process, concrete managerial ability and confidence in subordinates will prove to be the method of choice.[7]

REFERENCES

1. Rogers, V.L., and Lynch, J.J. "Coping Mechanisms Used by Hospital Middle Managers." *Topics in Health*

Record Management 6, no. 1 (1985): 36–43.
2. Veninga, R. "The Management of Disruptive

Conflicts." *Hospital and Health Services Administration* 24, no. 2 (1979): 8–29.

3. Guy, M.E. "Interdisciplinary Conflict and Organizational Complexity." *Hospital and Health Services Administration* 31, no. 1 (1986): 111–21.

4. Corwin, R. "Patterns of Organizational Conflict." *Administrative Science Quarterly* 12 (1979): 507–20.

5. Keane, A., Ducette, J., and Alder, D.C. "Stress in ICU and Non-ICU Nurses." *Nursing Research* 34, no. 4 (1985): 231–36.

6. Trunzo, T. "Group Conflict—A Challenge to Participative Management." *Hospital Topics* 63, no. 1 (1985): 36–37.

7. Cohen, A. "Tips to Improve the Manager/Leader's Performance." *Hospital Topics* 63, no. 1 (1985): 38–40.

Advantages and disadvantages of committees

I. Donald Snook, Jr.
President
Presbyterian–University of
Pennsylvania Medical Center
Philadelphia, Pennsylvania

HOW OFTEN HAS one heard "Let's turn this matter over to a committee," or "The committee recommends . . ." or "We need a committee to study this matter?" The use of committees is an organizational epidemic in America. However, committees are not solely an American tradition. Committees have their roots deep in Western civilization and the concept of using committees is associated with many of the common elements of democracy. Committees allow people to participate in decision making according to the "one man, one vote" principle.

People are taught early to work together on projects in school, in church, in communities and in other associations. In spite of the millions of committees that have been formed over the years, there still exists a certain degree of ambiguity and mystery about this management tool. One wonders, how should the committee

Health Care Superv, 1984,2(3),39–49
© 1984 Aspen Publishers, Inc.

be used? What are its disadvantages and its advantages? Committees can be a popular remedy for many administrative problems, or they can be a ploy to postpone decisions. At times committees end up being a true disaster for management. At one time or another, most of the major issues in most organizations will come through some type of committee. Committees are used at all levels in the organization.

WHAT IS A COMMITTEE?

A committee is a group of people who have been selected or otherwise brought together to deal with specific issues or problems of common interest. Where committees derive their authority varies from organization to organization. Often, being a committee member is a part-time job and a member will have principal duties in other areas of the organization. Committees frequently end up being decision-making groups, thereby affecting the work lives of others in the organization.

There are two kinds of committees: the standing or permanent committee and the ad hoc committee. The standing committee is usually described in the formal structure of the hospital or organization, perhaps in its bylaws or administrative policies and regulations. The scope, duties and authority of standing committees are generally well outlined. The ad hoc committee is formed for a specific purpose and usually has a well-defined, shorter life. These are temporary or special

purpose committees. It is common for ad hoc committees to collect and analyze data or to make specific recommendations to a higher authority. Ad hoc committees are often formed to search for candidates for key-position openings in the hospital. When used for this purpose they are called *search committees.*

PURPOSES OF COMMITTEES

If one queries why committees are so popular and why they continue to be used so regularly, the answer lies in the fact that they serve a growing number of purposes and meet an organization's needs. Managers display different biases about committees. Some like them; others feel they are useless. These mixed reviews are a clue to the fact that committees serve so many different purposes.

Two of the common purposes behind committees are that they bring a variety of minds together in a decision-making environment, and they use the "group-think" process to solve problems. In hospitals, committees have been quite important in problem solving, particularly since hospitals are made up of a diverse number of professionals and technicians working in the same environment in close contact. Hospital committees may have representation from a variety of different departments or functional areas in the institution. These individuals are brought together by management to solve problems not easily handled by one person.

Another function of committees, and an especially important one in health care organizations, is to help improve communications. Horizontal flow of information is important in hospitals. Committees offer an appropriate mechanism within America's highly departmentalized hospitals. Committees allow representatives from a variety of departments to sit down together and discuss common problems face to face. This type of communication is not easily achieved outside of committees.

Another key reason for establishing committees is to provide a means of recommending action to higher authority. The obvious advantage of a committee-recommended action is that it comes from a variety of people. Occasionally committees are set up for simple discussion only, along the lines of "Let's test the water on this matter," or "Let's find out what the group really thinks of this item." In hospitals, where there are so many different types of professionals and technicians with their own points of view, such discussion-only committees are common.

Occasionally committees are formed simply to collect information. In many instances this is the role of an ad hoc committee. Data may be collected orally or in writing. Committees may use a variety of techniques and devices to collect and sort information.

Making decisions and handing out sanctions is another key reason for forming committees. Also, committees offer a chance for peers in an or-

ganization to relate to each other. Committees can offer an excellent way to improve staff morale, give status to employees and build confidence in the individuals who participate.

Though there are a host of reasons to establish committees, perhaps the most important reason, at least in hospitals, is to bring individuals together to solve problems. When solving problems through committees the group must have a leader and a game plan. The key to a committee's success is planning. When a committee is successful in solving problems, other positive things happen in the hospital. When committees succeed in solving problems, morale is enhanced and the whole concept of team building takes on new meaning. This can be a valuable byproduct of successful committee action.

WHEN SHOULD COMMITTEES BE USED?

Management constantly faces the question, "When should we use a committee?" There are no hard and fast rules in answering this question. It is common for hospitals to have some standard committees. The medical staff, the board of trustees, administration and nursing service all use committees extensively. Committees may be used for planning, to work on budget problems, to review employee credentials or to discuss quality control issues. The list is almost endless. Not all hospitals use

Committees may be used for planning, to work on budget problems, to review employee credentials or to discuss quality control issues.

committees in the same way, nor do they have the same number and the same exact types of committees. Though it is dangerous to say exactly when a committee should be formed, some guidelines might be helpful. Some of the conditions that might lead an organization to use a committee are
- when there seems to be a divergence of data or opinions on a certain subject and one person would have some difficulty making a sound judgment;
- when a problem or a decision is of such major importance that it calls for several qualified persons to take a role in the decision-making or problem-solving process;
- when a problem or decision requires a broad-based appreciation or understanding of the issue, and when the input of a group of people would be advantageous;
- when different functions or departments are involved, and when obtaining positive results depends on securing the cooperation and successful coordination of much of the hospital staff.

HOW COMMITTEES FUNCTION BEST

To get the most out of a committee, it is wise to define the committee's scope and authority before it begins work. Such clarification will help the members immeasurably. Each committee should have a charge, that is, a defined scope, before starting work. If members are to offer ideas and recommendations, they should know to whom they are to make their recommendations. If they are to be responsible to another body or to another committee, they should know this as well. Incidentally, if the committee knows its limits it will help the committee members to evaluate its effectiveness.

Size should be considered when developing committees. It is important that committees be large enough to obtain solid discussion and input but not so large as to discourage dialogue or lead to indecision and inefficiency. A committee may be as small as 3 or 4 members or range upward to 12 to 15 members. Some organizations have found that 5 is an ideal committee size. With 5 there are enough members to spread the knowledge and skills, yet the committee is small enough to work efficiently. Larger numbers provide a broader base of skills but also mean that more time has to be given for allowing members to participate, which reduces the internal efficiency of the committee.

The role of the chairperson

It is no secret to one who has served on a committee that the chairperson is critical to the success of the committee's activities. An effective chairperson can increase the effectiveness of the whole body.

A chairperson should have a limited personal or professional stake in the committee's outcome or decision. The chairperson should be skillful in the art of arbitrating disputes and negotiating positions between different committee members. Patience must be the chairperson's companion. An effective chairperson must appear to be more neutral than negative or positive with the issues. The chairperson should be skillful in encouraging the correct balance of discussion, rather than necessarily allowing all discussion (which could lead the committee down false paths).

A successful chairperson should maintain a sense of humor. Being able to identify differences among committee members is also an important trait. There will be times when the chairperson must secure consensus on issues. Being a good timekeeper, ensuring that each committee member has a certain allotted time in which to contribute, can help the efficiency of the committee's work.

It is helpful for a chairperson to have a grasp of committee vocabulary. This person should be skillful in the use of jargon such as "Let's be sure we understand what we are implementing" or "Let's document this properly." The vocabulary and the psychology of words play an important role in a properly functioning committee. Such sentences as "My concern is . . . ," "Did I hear you say this?" or "Maybe you would like to rephrase that" all can be helpful. Words can remove barriers and add clarity to the committee's discussions.

The committee chairperson's main task is to control the committee's activities. If the chairperson fails in this role, the committee may go off in all directions and perhaps cause all members to be disappointed. The chairperson has the responsibility for sorting out the findings and results of committee activities and relating these to the committee's purpose. (But the leader has to be cautious and watch to see that the committee is not misled and does not become a refuge for someone's personal agenda items.) The committee chairperson has to know exactly what resources are available to the committee.

Much of the success of the committee function may depend on proper staff support. This could mean additional research, typing or administrative tasks. It is the chairperson's job to determine exactly what staff resources are available.

Finally, committees involve a group decision process or "group think," and it is important that the chairperson understand how to obtain consensus decisions from the membership. Consensus may not be a clear-cut win or lose situation. By using consensus a skillful chairperson can create cohesiveness in a group and avoid divisiveness.

The agenda

It usually falls to the chairperson to create an agenda for each meeting. The agenda can be a powerful tool and a driving force before, during and after each meeting. The agenda can give focus and order to the meeting.

Often it is necessary to set time limits on agenda items. Agenda items should be prioritized, the most important coming first and the least important near the end. It is helpful for the chairperson to place names next to each item. This allows members to prepare in advance. Some chairpersons like the approach of starting a meeting with a review, bringing the committee members up to date on the committee's activities. This is especially important if the committee has been meeting sporadically or if a good deal of time has elapsed between meetings.

Successful chairpeople remember to distribute the agenda a reasonable time in advance of the meeting. It is embarrassing for a chairperson to arrive at a meeting and see that the members have not received the agenda in advance.

The hidden agenda

Formal agendas are organized, typed, distributed and usually fairly well understood, but there may be other informal items within a "hidden agenda." The hidden agenda may be representative of the real give and take among committee members. It may be politics, power struggles, issues of leadership or a host of other items. Hidden agendas may be loaded with emotion and charged with excitement. Hidden agendas may be discussed between committee members well in advance of the meeting and are often unrelated to the formal agenda items.

One should not be surprised if the hidden agendas become the real business of some committees. Sophisticated committee members realize that these exist and must be dealt with. One clue that a hidden agenda might be taking over is when a committee seems to have the simple, straightforward issue on the table, yet it takes much longer to discuss and to get resolution than would seem to be necessary. Frequently it falls to the chairperson to search out and understand hidden agendas and lead the committee through them. It is both the committee's job and the chairperson's job to proceed with the agenda, not to allow hidden agendas to subvert the purpose of the group.

A committee member's role

There is no "ideal" committee member. A committee's work, like a fine meal, has to be balanced and well thought out. The exact number and background of the people serving are best guided by the committee's purpose. If the committee's objective is to make strategic recommendations for the hospital, perhaps a high-level management group should be dominant rather than technical personnel. If the committee is out to win friends and influence minds on an issue, then perhaps committee members should be selected for their natural leadership abilities. The position of various committee members in the informal as well as the formal organization should be considered. If the committee's role is to compromise what appears to be a difficult situation, then one must look for individuals with negotiating skills and middle-of-the-road personalities. If the committee is to be a final decision-making body on a weighty or controversial issue, one might look for an illustrious group of individuals whose judgment in the past has been unquestioned. The specific type of committee member depends on the committee's purposes.

Staff assistance

The work of a committee and its members can be made considerably easier if the role of its staff assistants is well planned. Some committees may meet often and be very active. This may mean that a great deal of research and homework must be done. It is unfair and unproductive to ask the chairperson to act as the committee secretary or to handle other staff tasks. The committee and its chairperson have a responsibility to request, and even demand, appropriate staff assistance. This may mean the group is assigned a full- or part-time secretary, a research assistant or whatever other assistance is necessary to accomplish the job. Effective staff assistants can keep in touch with committee members, make sure agendas are distributed, act as focal points for committee members who have questions, gather information or perform a host of other housekeeping details prior to meetings. They can also be invaluable as time savers for both the committee and its members. Proper staff assistance can greatly enhance the committee's final product.

ADVANTAGES OF COMMITTEES

By allowing greater participation by members, properly selected, well-balanced committees can produce better, more rational decisions. This may be the most valuable advantage of committees. The participation process is much more than saying, "Two heads are better than one." Proper committee work is a matter of pooling, mixing and blending the proper personalities and ideas in a group forum. To paraphrase the great English essayist Thomas Carlyle, a counting of heads does not make the truth. The best committees are synergistic; they blend opinions and intellects. One plus one often comes out something greater than two. Committees allow thoughts to be added to each other, not subtracted.

When a committee's objective is action, it is up to the group to enlist support for the action. Committees can be invaluable in securing cooperative effort. It is generally accepted that people who have a degree of responsibility for making decisions and have to carry out those decisions realize that securing support of key people in the organizations will make the decisions more lasting and more successful. This is why many executives look to committees to secure cooperation and consensus. The committee itself may go out into the organization and help sell the recommendations to others either formally or informally.

When positions in the organization seem to be frozen at opposite ends of the pole, a committee can be helpful in sidetracking emotions. A committee can offer a forum in which the parties can ventilate. In this regard a committee can be an excellent vehicle for cooling tempers. Management continues to use committees to divert volatile emotional issues and buy time for the organization to work out solutions.

Hospitals and other health care organizations are subject to constant stress and endless change. Any successful organization must have a continuity of ideas that guides it. This usually comes from top management. Turnover within top management through termination, promotion or retirement can disturb this continuity. Committees can play a major role in cementing the continuity of ideas within an organization, especially in this fast-paced, changing hospital world where the need is great for decisive planning and action. Hospital committees can provide a more lasting degree of continuity beyond what one individual can offer.

Many organizations conduct their work almost entirely through committees. Organizations that function through committees routinely place more junior members on committees shortly after they join the management or supervisory team. Members are "paying their dues" by serving their time in apprenticeship roles. Committee assignments can be a valuable training ground for employees, department heads, middle managers and top executives. Serving on committees is a way to develop management in the organization. Supervisors and department heads have an opportunity to watch management role models first hand. They have an opportunity to see and participate in the decision-making process. They can test their own people skills. They have an opportunity to be assigned staff work outside their own functional areas. Committee participation can give insight and a broader view to the manager of a technical department. Using committees as a means to develop personnel should not be overlooked as one of the major advantages of committees.

DISADVANTAGES OF COMMITTEES

When the organization is anxiously awaiting a firm recommendation or decision, committees often continue to move at their own pace and may add much more time to the process than an individual would. To people in the organization it may seem that committee action is always stalled.

Some techniques employed to reduce lost time include seeing that meetings are arranged well in advance and making sure that they are scheduled at regular times. Meeting dates are then placed on everyone's calendar. This will not guarantee that time will be saved, but it is a proven way of making a committee more efficient.

Even if committees meet regularly, their members show up punctually and there are few absences, committees are people organizations and their nature is to use up many personnel hours. Hospitals are costly, labor-intensive organizations, and committees add to the cost of hospital decision making. The cost is not simply calculated by adding together each participant's hourly wage. There is also the opportunity cost. If all the hours spent in committee actions were spent on some other project or activity, what would have been gained? Presumably in some cases the alternative would have been productive. Another factor to be weighed is the nature of people and how they deal with the many hours before and after the formal committee meetings. Committee members may spend a considerable amount of time before and after each meeting rediscussing agenda items. This is yet another time loss and thereby a cost to the organization.

Taken individually, employees may be responsible workers, but when they come together in a committee there can be a "thinning" of responsibility and a lessening of the

feeling of being held accountable. This is a natural consequence of group decisions. If an individual is

---

Taken individually, employees may be responsible workers, but when they come together in a committee there can be a "thinning" of responsibility and a lessening of the feeling of being held accountable.

---

asked to solve a problem or make a recommendation as part of a committee's decision, there is another kind of pressure. The dilution of responsibility through divided accountability can sometimes hinder management. Some of the characteristics of committees that share responsibility include rendering both a majority and a minority report, or stressing form and process over outcome; or being more concerned with agenda items, the democratic process and efficiency rather than outcome. There is only so much pressure for accountability that an organization can bring to bear on a chairperson to counter these tendencies. The net result is that it is difficult to hold committees accountable for group decisions.

One of the more frustrating times in committee work occurs when an individual feels he or she knows the proper way the organization should move on a topic or issue but the committee, through the democratic process and the give and take of ideas, offers a watered-down, compromise solution. The feeling that a compromise solution is wrong or unworkable may lead to a minority committee report.

A word about the minority report is in order. If the committee's primary role is advisory and it is asked to make a recommendation, the minority report might be helpful to management. On the other hand, if the committee is asked to render a solid, clean, crisp decision, the minority report could cause management problems in carrying out the decision. (The chairperson and the committee members should be on guard against using the vote too liberally. Sometimes voting can intimidate members, especially if the vote is called for too early. Arriving at a consensus without a vote might allow for less intimidation.)

Committees, like some employees, can become stagnated. Employees who become stagnated and nonproductive are called "dead wood." Perhaps the stagnated committees could be called a pile of dead wood. Committees, like products, have a life cycle (or a use cycle). It is management's job to evaluate committees and understand where they are in their life cycles. At the proper time, management may have to stop investing the organization's resources into a given committee. Committees may have to be abandoned or folded into other committees. This is particularly important for hospitals, more now than in the past. Times are changing rapidly, and if committees fail to

change, this may signal the organization's failure to keep up with the change.

EVALUATING COMMITTEES

There are some who recommend that each committee in the organization, including those of the medical staff and the board of trustees, be formally reviewed every few years by a team consisting of members from administration, the board and the medical staff. Such a review is healthy for an organization. Committees must be willing to change direction in order to presume their value. This kind of vitality is necessary for an effective committee.

ALBATROSS OR CATALYST?

A committee can be an albatross around the organization's neck, or it can be a catalyst in getting things done and creating new ideas. There are legitimate reasons for both using and avoiding using committees. Committees can help accomplish difficult tasks, or they can stall recommendations and delay action. Committees can set clear-cut objectives and meet them, or they can become process-oriented, costly exercises. Committees can solve difficult problems, or they can primarily be forums for power demonstrations and the exercise of political strength in the organization.

Committees can be all of these things. Which committees are warranted and needed is a management determination. Mature management has learned that committees are not always going to work, but they are valuable administrative tools which, when properly structured and monitored, can be extremely useful to the organization.

SUGGESTED READINGS

Newman, W.H. *Administrative Action.* Englewood Cliffs, NJ: Prentice-Hall, 1950.

Marriner, A. "Behavioral Aspects of Decision Making." *Supervisor Nurse* 8 (March 1977): 40–47.

Monson, T. "Mastering the Art of Planning by Committee." *Journal of Nursing Administration* 11 (November–December 1981): 71–72.

Walton, M. "Just a Part of the Routine." *Nursing Mirror* 150 (January 1980): 32–34.

"Nursing Committees Participate in Management." *Hospital Progress* 63 (August 1982): 52–53.

"Committee Plan Helps Resolve Problems Between Department." *Hospitals* 56 (July 1982): 61–67.

Topham, A.S. "Medical Staff Committees Benefit from Job Description." *The Hospital Medical Staff* 11 (November 1982): 22–25.

Williams, K.J., and Donnelly, P.R. "How to Make Committees Work for You." *The Hospital Medical Staff* 11 (May 1982): 6–11.

How to generate power
in meetings

William Umiker
Adjunct Clinical Professor
Pathology Department
Pennsylvania State University
Hershey, Pennsylvania

PROFESSIONALS AND managers spend much of their time at meetings. This time expenditure increases as one moves up in an organization. Although many meetings are time wasters that often end in frustration, important decisions are made in that setting. Therefore, it behooves us to be effective when serving on committees or task forces or participating in staff meetings, budget conferences, and other assemblages.

PREPARATION AND ARRIVAL

If you do not receive an agenda or if the purpose of the meeting is unclear, ask for more information. This shows that you are interested and enables you to be better prepared. You may want to contact the leader to ask if there are any special data or reports you should bring.

Arrive on time so you do not miss anything that could adversely affect your objectives or

Health Care Superv, 1990, 9(1), 33–38
©1990 Aspen Publishers, Inc.

proposals. If the meeting does not start promptly, use the opportunity for networking. This time also provides a good opportunity to test the waters regarding any proposals you may be considering.

Stand near the door and greet people, but do not upstage the moderator. Introduce yourself to any new members. Do not sit in a corner and look forlorn.

ASSERTIVENESS IS OF FUNDAMENTAL IMPORTANCE

A high level of self-esteem is essential to one's ability to garner support and be persuasive. Nonassertive individuals suffer from a chronic deficiency of self-esteem, and therefore lack power in group meetings.

Assertiveness training via seminars and educational courses can be effective, and these programs are available in most locations. However, many shy people are afraid to enroll in them because they fear the role-playing and confrontational exercises that are involved. Books and audiotapes on assertiveness, while less effective, are still worthwhile.

There are two effective tactics for nonassertive individuals to use at meetings. The first is *escalating dialogue*, in which the passive member breaks the ice by asking questions. The initial questions are benign requests for information or for clarification, followed by more challenging queries, and finally, comments and suggestions.

The second is to maintain a state of *interested and active neutrality* during controversies. Opposing members try to convince the fence sitter, who then becomes a center of attention. Simply listening to both sides and asking appropriate questions provides the neutral observer with clout.

GENERATE POWER THROUGH YOUR ACTIONS AND REACTIONS

Words

Try to generate power from words. For example, try the following:

- Use the other person's name frequently. One's name is one's favorite word.
- Avoid discounters like "I know this sounds silly, but..." or "I know you will laugh when you hear...." Discounters are self–put-downs.
- Avoid weasel words like "maybe" or "I'll try." Substitute strong statements like "let's do it..." instead of "maybe we should...." (except in the tentative phase of confronting, as is discussed later in this article).
- Avoid cliches like "it goes without saying" or "it happens to the best of us."
- Avoid fillers like "ya know" or "Uhhhhhh."

Delivery

Generate power from your delivery by sounding enthusiastic; speaking clearly and forcefully, making one point at a time; and not tolerating repeated interruptions. Interruptions short-circuit influence and bash self-esteem. Just say, "Harry, I was not finished" and keep talking. Do not wait for an apology. It may not be forthcoming, thus adding to your embarrassment.

Listening

Listening is crucial. The more you know what is going on, the greater the advantage you have. Being the best listener in most groups is not difficult; usually only a few participants are really listening. The others are talking, daydreaming, or mentally script writing (thinking of what they are going to say). Listen for facts and for feelings. Listen for what is *not* being said. Listen with your eyes. Watch facial expressions, gestures,

---

Listen for facts and for feelings.
Listen for what is **not** *being said.*

---

and other body language of the senders and the receivers. Over 50% of the impact of verbal communication comes from this sign language.

Body language

Work on improving your skill at interpreting body communication. Frowns, smiles, winks, and nods send clear messages. Others can be more subtle: For instance, can you recognize the six different emotions that are revealed in facial expressions? They are surprise, fear, anger, disgust, happiness, and sadness.

Raising an eyebrow, rubbing the nose, or folding the arms across the chest are sure signs of disbelief or disagreement. When people suddenly look upwards and rapidly blink their eyes, they are giving serious consideration to what you said. When they lean forward, touch or rub their chins, nod their heads and smile, they approve. If you see the moderator tapping the table with a pencil, tugging on an ear, or shifting restlessly, it is time to stop talking.

Watch out for mixed messages. A *mixed message* is one in which the words say something different than do the phonetics, voice tone, facial expression, or other body language. Body language is much more powerful than words and usually delivers the true message. Steve may say that he is pleased with a decision, but his voice cracks, he frowns, and his fingers grow restless.

Do not deliver mixed messages, and challenge other people when they do. In the above scenario, an appropriate remark would be "Steve, you say that you're pleased with this decision, but your expression suggests otherwise. How do you really feel about this?"

Beware of hidden communication. Statements often have dual contents. A surface message is factual or plausible, whereas a hidden communication is a barb aimed at the listener's ego. For example, a chairperson might respond to a member's suggestion with the plausible message, "Louise, I can't accept that idea," followed by "I am surprised that you would suggest that." The hidden message is "Louise, you're an idiot." Hidden messages damage interpersonal relationships and should be avoided unless the second message is complimentary.

When you are on the receiving end of a negative hidden communication, do not let the remark pass without comment, because it will encourage the speaker to deliver more hidden messages or make direct attacks. Louise should respond with "Ann, just what did you mean by that remark?" Now Ann must either deny a secondary message or confirm it for what it was.

You can generate power from positions and body language, as well. For example, try the following:

- Sit next to your antagonist, not across from him or her. When you address that person, turn 30 degrees toward the person instead of merely turning your head.
- Maintain a column of air between your back and the back of your chair. Leaning forward shows interest.

- Expand your personal space. Spread out a little. Move your arms away from your body. Resting forearms on the table expands personal space and projects power. Place some papers in front of you. Do not restrict your personal space by crossing your arms on your lap. When you use minimal space, your message is "I am not important."
- Gestures indicate power: Vary them. To project confidence, for instance, join the fingertips of both hands in a steepling fashion.
- Stand when talking. Power varies directly with eye-level variances. Place a hand on your hip when you are registering a strong negative response.
- Smile at the right time. It has been said that people who smile *when pleased* have power. People who smile *to please* lack it.
- Maintain eye contact, but do not stare.

NEGOTIATION AND CONFRONTATION

How to respond to other peoples' ideas

Encourage suggestions, or at least be open to them. Use the "PIN" approach: State what you regard as the *P*ositive aspects of an idea. If there are none, say that it is *I*nteresting. React to the *N*egative aspects last. When you agree with others, support their ideas enthusiastically. Try to build on their suggestions.

When you disagree with another, do it amicably. Phrase your critique in the form of concerns or possible limitations. Before you do, be sure that you comprehend the person's argument. Question in a nonthreatening way, ask open-ended questions, and paraphrase the speaker's comments to ensure clarity.

How to get your points across

Be prepared. Have your proposal well-organized: This includes rehearsing your opening and closing statements. Write out a specific motion before or during the meeting. Consider all the possible objections and how you will respond to each.

Try to visualize a highly successful presentation. This exercise, called *performance imagery,* has been used very successfully by athletes, salespersons, and speakers. Also, apply the verbal and behavioral suggestions described earlier during your presentation. If you run into opposition, use confrontational strategy.

How to confront

Hear your opponents out

When people take vigorous exception to your proposal, question, or comment, hold your fire until you have heard and comprehended exactly what their objections are. Do not interrupt, even if they make untrue or

---

When individuals are upset, both sending and receiving may be flawed.

---

inflammatory statements. It is essential that you understand not only their viewpoints, but also their feelings. Maintain your composure: If you become defensive or distraught, you will be at a distinct disadvantage.

Ask for clarification if the message you get is garbled. When individuals are upset, both sending and receiving may be flawed. Paraphrase what was said. Do not be surprised if you hear "No, no, that's not at all what I said. I said ...."

Use *negative inquiry* to get at the root of criticism. For example, in a nonsarcastic tone say, "I don't understand. Exactly what is it about my statement that bothers you?" "There must be more; what else bothers you?" "Was it the way I said it that annoyed you?"

Respond tentatively

Be diplomatic. Use conditional terminology like "it sounds as though" or "possibly." Express your points in the form of suggestions or motions, not demands. Make your statements as palatable as possible: "Lois, you present a convincing argument, I have to hand it to you. However, I'm still of the opinion that...."

Try fogging or negative assertion to defuse antagonists. *Fogging* is agreeing with part of what they said: "You're right, I often do come up with harebrained ideas, but I don't think this is one of them." Negative assertion is accepting some blame, saying something like, "That was a dumb thing I did."

Reinforce areas of agreement. When people state things with which you agree, smile and nod. When you disagree, present an expressionless countenance.

Switch to firm confrontation if the tentative approach fails

Keep your voice low, slow, and measured: talking faster, louder, or at a higher pitch escalates conflict. Do not attack people; address what they said or did. The easiest way to achieve this is to switch from "you" language to "I" language. Instead of "You get me very upset when you say that," say "I get very upset when I hear such statements."

Avoid absolute words like "never" or "always" and inflammatory ones like "you have to," "you're wrong," or "I demand." Avoid also the use of "why" questions when you really mean "you shouldn't have." For example, "Why do you continue to repeat these half-truths?" really means, "You shouldn't have continued to say that."

Avoid put-downs like "Let's get back to reality," "You can't be serious," or "We'd be a laughing stock." Also, avoid threatening gestures like finger pointing, fist shaking, scowling, or sneering.

Use an escape statement

If you think you have lost the encounter and compromise is not likely, make a statement like, "Alice, this argument is making me very uncomfortable. Could we continue discussing this at another time?"

WIN ARGUMENTS WITHOUT LOSING FRIENDS

In the ideal resolution of a confrontation, both parties get what they want. However, such win-win situations are often not possible. Unfortunately, a win-loss encounter sets you up for a loss later. Your opponent withdraws to regroup or to fight back indirectly. If you can compromise without losing too much, it is often better than going for the jugular.

Sometimes it is possible to let a loser down gently by using the "3-F" strategy proposed by Salzman.[1] The three Fs are "Feel," "Felt," and "Find." Suppose you have had an argument with your students over a new schedule. Here is how you could end the discussion.

- "I know you all *feel* very strongly about this: I can understand that" (empathy).
- "Last year's class *felt* just as you do now" (misery loves company).

- "I'm certain that a month from now you'll *find* you prefer the new schedule" (happy ending).

• • •

Planning, active listening, and assertiveness are prerequisites for getting the results you want at meetings. Shy members may find escalating dialogue and active neutrality helpful in participating more effectively in groups. Maximum individual power is generated by judicious selection of words, forceful delivery, and emphatic body language.

REFERENCE

1. Salzman, J. "How to Get Results with People." Boulder, Colo.: CareerTrack Publishers, 1987. Sound cassette.

Running small meetings:
An overlooked technique for making them productive and keeping them short

Marianna Nelson, B.S.N., M.A.
Research Coordinator
Newington Children's Hospital

Zane Saunders, M.A.
Former Director of Speech Pathology and
*   Audiology*
Former Chair, Institutional Review Board
Newington Children's Hospital
Newington, Connecticut

ARTICLES about improving the way meetings are run emphasize group dynamics, especially the leader's role in diverting and handling personalities and interactions that can affect meetings in unproductive or negative ways.[1-4] Although two of these articles[1,2] also discuss using agenda or other means to set up a format and goals, none describe how to use Robert's Rules of Order to run meetings. If they did, probably few people would read them because of an intimidating mystique that surrounds the rules. This stems from the complexity of the original source, *Robert's Rules of Order, Newly Revised,*[5] and the formal language used in parliamentary procedure guides such as those intended for a national assembly where delegates face skilled opponents.[6,7] These sources are cumbersome and difficult to use as quick reference tools and lack the information necessary to guide a leader who is dissatisfied with loosely run smaller meetings and who wants to change. How unfortunate this is. As a result, Robert's Rules of

Health Care Superv, 1992, 11(1), 68–75
©1992 Aspen Publishers, Inc.

Order have become underused and unappreciated at most small meetings. Furthermore, there are fewer chairpersons who know how to use the rules correctly and who can serve as role models for others.

When the rules are used fully and correctly, however, the need for leaders to be personality facilitators and mediators is greatly diminished. The structure of the rules frees the chairperson from the constant responsibility of keeping discussions on track or directing them back on track. In fact, it was for these reasons that the rules were written. In 1867, Henry Martyn Robert,[5] who was an army major at the time, was transferred to San Francisco where he and his wife joined local groups to try to improve social conditions. Their meetings were attended by vocal new settlers who had conflicting ideas. Even though Robert tried to settle disputes and bring order, these took much of his time and effort and he felt the groups were not accomplishing as much as they could. He began to study manuals on parliamentary law and adapted them into rules he could use at his meetings. Over time he refined and expanded these rules into a flexible tool that has been recognized for many years as the standard for organizations and clubs.

The rules provide a structure for any group to express its ideas and then to find solutions that reflect the will within the whole membership. Additional benefits are that meetings become shorter and more productive without jeopardizing the spirit that is vital to small groups. Also, the minutes are easier to write because the meeting procedures make clear what was discussed and what decisions were made.

The purpose of this article is to remove the mystery and formality from Robert's Rules of Order and describe a strategy for switching to the rules and sticking with them. Since June 1988, the steps, procedures, and tips described in this article (see box) have been successfully used by the Institutional Review Board (IRB) for research at Newington Children's Hospital and can be applied to most other committees and boards.

The IRB, a standing committee that meets about seven times a year, has grown from nine members in 1988 when it first started

---

Steps for Making the Change and Making It Stick

- Announce the change, institute it, then celebrate!
- Familiarize members with basics of correct use:
  — propose a motion first, then discuss it
  — reserve a special time during the meeting when other comments can be heard; these have the potential for becoming motions at future meetings.
- Ask individual members to prepare specific motions.
- Base each agenda on the order of business for meetings (see other box).
- Provide a brief orientation for new members.

- Think of Robert as the meeting monitor.
- Refer to motions (not their makers) through the chair.
- If rules are modified, make sure:
  — everyone knows what the changes are
  — the new rules are used consistently.
- Learn correct use of the rules:
  — observe the rules in use, especially at meetings of local government commissions and councils
  — read about the rules
- Encourage and teach others correct use and show the benefits of meetings run with Robert's Rules of Order.

using the rules to 17 members in 1991. The Board was established in 1984 to review and approve research proposals according to standards for human subject protection established by the Department of Health and Human Services and according to guidelines and procedures that the board itself has set up and refined over the years.[8–10]

MAKE THE CHANGE SMOOTHLY AND MAKE IT STICK

First meeting: Announce the change, institute it, then celebrate!

The best time to introduce the new structure is at a meeting for which the agenda is short. Our agenda was very short the first time; in fact, what we needed to do probably could have waited for another meeting. Yet, because of this, it was an opportune time to introduce the new procedures. It also gave us time to celebrate. We had arranged for the Food Service Department to send an English high tea to the meeting room; by making the first meeting a big occasion in this way, it was memorable and has set the precedent for a celebration of some sort each year.

The main objectives of the first meeting are to announce that meetings will be run by Robert's Rules of Order and to explain the three key changes, as follows:

(1) after an agenda is introduced, the motion related to it must be made before the discussion can begin;

(2) general comments not related to a motion or order of business can be discussed at a designated time later in the meeting; and

(3) meeting agenda will be organized according to the order of business (see box).

Order of Business for Meetings

I. Reading and approval of minutes from last meeting

II. Correspondence
   A. Incoming
   B. Outgoing

III. Reports of ad hoc committees

IV. Special orders

V. Unfinished business

VI. New business

VII. Announcements

VIII. For the good of the board. This is an opportunity for members to make general comments that do not need a formal motion.

Adapted from *Robert's Rules of Order, Newly Revised.* Glenview, Ill.: Scott, Foresman, 1970.

Not following the first two rules presents the greatest deterrent to efficiency. Unrelated conversations can easily work their way into discussions, causing delays and also putting an unnecessary burden on the chairperson to direct the discussion back to the agenda item. Making a motion first, however, channels the discussion and helps to keep it on track so the leader does not have to continually focus the members' energy and attention on the discussion. If discussion does stray, it is very effective if the chair says, for example, "We're discussing a motion to add a new procedure for review of research protocols."

Making a motion before discussing it will seem strange at first, since the opposite order is followed at most small meetings. This change will be accepted readily, however, when the group sees firsthand that meetings are shorter and productivity is greatly improved. Acceptance continues to increase with members' assurance that whatever they wish to present to the others can and will be heard at the proper time.

How can a group become familiar enough with a subject without discussing it before a motion is made? One way to accomplish this is for the chair to assign an item of business to a member and give that person the responsibility of making a motion related to it. Any initial timidity about making a formal main motion usually disappears with encouragement from the chairperson before the meeting or by help with phrasing or rephrasing a motion for clarity at the meeting.

At our meetings, assignments work like this: at least two weeks before a meeting a primary reviewer is assigned to review a research proposal that is in his or her area of expertise. At the meeting, the reviewer summarizes and evaluates the proposal and then makes a motion according to one of the three options the board has established: to approve the proposal as submitted, approve it with stipulations, or reject it and give guidelines for revision. With this procedure, a motion flows naturally from the reviewer's presentation and the discussion and voting processes are greatly expedited.

Adopt agenda and follow it consistently

The agenda, which is organized according to the order of business, is sent out about two weeks before each meeting. It serves as a periodic reminder of a group's commitment to using the rules and gives a consistent structure and organization to all the meetings. The agenda should contain a list of all the correspondence and other items, routine and nonroutine, to keep members well informed. Including all items on the agenda

and going through them at the meeting is well worth the extra time.

Familiarize members with basics of correct use

Because many people either have never used the rules at all or have had no opportunity to use them fully or correctly, the overall goal is to have members become familiar and at ease with using rules the right way. At a brief orientation held with each new member individually, the chairperson explains how the rules are used. At smaller meetings, it is likely that only a few basic rules will be needed but it is important that every member know which rules they are and how they work. Also, changes in procedure can be made but any changes must be introduced, understood, and consistently used.

The more the rules are used, the better they work. After a few meetings, members learn to anticipate the order of business and the sequence of motions and they become at ease with the structure. With this comes the realization of the many benefits of using the rules.

Think of Robert as meeting monitor

Robert has become an invisible, advisory member of our board. This means that Robert and his rules, not us, are blamed if, for example, someone forgets and brings up comments unrelated to the discussion. In addition, because the correct procedure for discussing or debating a motion is for mem-

Movers and seconders of motions are not bound to vote in favor of the motions they made.

bers to direct their comments through the chair rather than each other directly and to disagree by referring to the motion rather than the person who made it, the potential for problems arising from disagreements is greatly reduced.[11]

Role of the chairperson

Be prepared

A well-prepared leader goes over the agenda before each meeting, regarding it as a script with a changeable plot in which the actors determine the direction the plot will take. Therefore, the well-prepared leader will know each agenda item well, will anticipate in advance the different directions each discussion might take, and will be ready to offer comments if needed.

A good leader always knows the right thing to say at meetings but says it only if no one else does. If reaching a decision is imminent but eludes the group, the cognizant leader can make the group's choice become more apparent by restating points already made or by asking key questions. Because the rules have removed most of the chair's burden of policing meetings, leaders are more free to direct their time and energy in this way.

In his article, "The Meeting Chairperson: Master or Servant?," Jay sums up the chairperson's position and responsibilities as follows. If as chairperson,

> . . . you are to make sure that the meeting achieves valuable objectives, you will be more effective seeing yourself as the servant of the group rather than as its master. Your role then becomes to assist the group toward the best conclusion or decision in the most efficient manner possible: to interpret and clarify, to move the discussion forward, and to bring it to a resolution that everyone understands and accepts as being the will of the meeting, even if individuals do not necessarily agree with it.[12(p.30)]

Avoid manipulating meetings

Rules of order of any kind can be used to manipulate meetings. However, if meeting rules are used as intended, a real participatory democracy will reign. This effectively reduces autocratic control not only of the chair but also of the biggest mouth.

Jay[12] remarks that one of the best and most effective chairpersons he has served under intervenes in a discussion with only one sentence, or at the most, two. One would assume that this self-imposed restriction greatly reduces the risk of manipulation taking hold and gives the leader more time to analyze and evaluate what the members are saying.

The chairperson's manner

A smooth transition to meetings run entirely by Robert's Rules of Order depends not only on the chairperson's skill and knowledge in the use of the rules but also on the demeanor of the chairperson. A calm, confident manner and a resonant voice all help in getting members to accept and appreciate the structure.

HOW MOTIONS WORK

The way motions work is based on logic, good sense, and fair play.[6,7] Making a main motion is a mechanism for getting an item of business on the floor so that it can be discussed and then voted on in such a way that the will of the majority will prevail in the decision. Thus making a motion does not mean that it will be passed as stated, or even passed at all; however, if this is handled in an impersonal way as discussed above, such a decision will not be a reflection against any member of the group. Movers and seconders of motions are not bound to vote in favor of

the motions they made. They have the obligation, just as the other members do, to be open-
minded during discussion and therefore they
have the right to change their minds.[11]

The next four sections illustrate how some
motions work.

A main motion and amendments

Assume that a primary reviewer summarizes and evaluates a research proposal and
then makes a motion to approve the proposal
with specific stipulations about the consent
form. Another member seconds the motion.
The motion to approve and each stipulation
are restated by the chair and recorded by the
person taking the minutes. During the discussion another member points out weaknesses
in the proposal itself and recommends
changes. One way to handle this situation is
for a member to amend the main motion with
new stipulations for the proposal. The
amendment is also seconded and then it is
accepted by the chair. The new stipulations
are recorded and the amendment is discussed. After the amendment is voted on, if it
passes, the chair calls for a vote of the main
motion in its amended form; if the amendment does not pass, the chair calls for a vote
on the original main motion.[5] In either case,
the last step is for the chair to announce the
results of voting.

Amendments give flexibility to the rules
and are probably the most widely used of the
subsidiary motions.[5] It is important to remember that amendments are made for the
purpose of improving an original motion;
they cannot reverse its intent, such as by
adding the word "not." Although Robert[5]
says that amendments can be amended,
Perry[11] in his interpretation of the rules says
they cannot. For the sake of keeping small
meetings simple, perhaps this is good advice.

Also, there cannot be more than one amendment on the floor at a time.

Division of a question

Dividing a question facilitates discussion
and voting when there is more than one part,
as in the case of the research proposal described above. It is preferable to divide the
main question when it is first introduced but
it can be done at any time. In the example,
dividing the question will result in one motion about the consent form and another
about the proposal; each question is handled
separately and treated as an individual motion.[5,11]

Withdrawing a motion

When it appears that an original motion has
lost support, its maker can request permission from the chair to withdraw the motion.
Once the motion has been accepted (restated)
by the chair, it no longer is the property of its
maker; it belongs to the group and cannot be
withdrawn or altered by the mover or sec-
onder without permission.[5] (It can be withdrawn without permission, however, before
it is accepted by the chair). In a situation in
which the original motion has lost support,
Perry[11] recommends that it is best disposed of
by the chair calling for the vote and moving
on.

A motion to reconsider

Groups, just like the individuals, change
their minds. It is for this reason that the rules
include a motion to reconsider. This allows a
group to change its mind one time only about
a motion as long as the motion has not been
acted on. (This rule does not apply to a
motion to adjourn.) If the group's change of
mind is about a motion that was passed or
defeated at a previous meeting, the motion to

reconsider can be moved, seconded, accepted, and passed in the usual way. Occasionally it may concern a motion from the same meeting. In this case, the mover of the motion to reconsider must be a member who voted with the majority on the original vote.[5,11]

RESOURCES

Table 1 gives the requirements of some of the more frequently used parliamentary motions. If a question arises during meetings about how to handle a motion, using this

Table 1. Requirements of some more frequently used parliamentary motions.

The motion	Precedence of motion	Second for motion	Discussion of motion	Amendment to motion	Vote on motion
Main motion	Only when nothing is pending	Yes	Yes	Yes	Majority
Subsidiary motions:					
Table	In	Yes	Yes	Yes (limited)	Majority
Amend	descending	Yes	Yes	Yes	Majority
Refer	order	Yes	Yes	Yes	Majority
Limit discussion		Yes	No	Yes	2/3
Call previous question		Yes	No	No	2/3
Incidental motions:					
Suspend rules	In	Yes	No	No	2/3
Withdraw motion	descending order	No	No	No	Without objection
Point of order		No	No	No	Chair
Appeal from chair		Yes	No	No	Majority
Divide question		No	No	Yes	Majority
Privileged motions:					
Point of privilege	In	No	No	No	Chair
Recess	descending	Yes	No	Yes	Majority
Adjourn	order	Yes	No	No (limited)	Majority
Motion that brings a question again before the assembly:					
Reconsider	Takes precedence to nothing over all; yields	Yes	When applied to a debatable motion	No	Majority

table enables the chair or other person to find the answer quickly. Note that the table indicates that a main motion can be made only when no other motion is pending. Furthermore, subsidiary, privileged, and certain incidental motions can be made while a main motion is pending.[5] Although it may seem surprising that a main motion has the lowest rank of all and has to yield to all other motions, this is because many other motions can affect a main motion and therefore it has to be voted on last.

Three pamphlets,[13–15] one article,[16] and three books[11,17,18] are clearly written and can help one become familiar with the system. Because the original rules were written over one hundred years ago, adaptation and interpretations have been made and, therefore, some differences do exist between the newer sources and the original.

• • •

Those who have learned the rules and appreciate their benefits have a responsibility to lead others and encourage them to use the rules at their meetings. Consistent use will enable small groups to accomplish more with seemingly less effort and also will help them to make informed, careful decisions as they face complex challenges in the health care field today.

REFERENCES

1. Haynes, M.E. "How To Conduct Quality Meetings." *Clinical Laboratory Management Review* (January/February 1990): 29–36.
2. Jay, A. "How to Run a Meeting." *Journal of Nursing Administration* (January 1982): 22–8.
3. Lancaster, J. "Making the Most of Meetings." *Journal of Nursing Administration* (October 1981): 15–9.
4. Mosel, D. "Communications Workshop. How To Evaluate—and Enhance—Your Meeting." *Voluntary Action Leadership* (Fall 1981): 18–20.
5. Robert, H.M. *Robert's Rules of Order, Newly Revised.* Glenview, Ill.: Scott, Foresman, 1970.
6. "How to Use Parliamentary Procedure." *Association of Operating Room Nurses Journal* 43, no. 1 (1986): 155–164.
7. "A Guide on Parliamentary Procedure." *Association of Operating Room Nurses Journal* 47, no. 1 (1988): 97–105.
8. Department of Health and Human Services, Office for Protection from Research Risks. *Code of Federal Regulations, Title 45—Public Welfare, Part 46—Protection of Human Subjects.* Washington, D.C.: Government Printing Office, 1983.
9. Newington Children's Hospital, Institutional Review Board. "Quantitative Research Proposal Guide; Qualitative Research Proposal Guide." Revised August 1990.
10. Newington Children's Hospital, Institutional Review Board. *Procedures Manual.* Revised June 1990.
11. Perry, H. *Call To Order.* Burlington, Ontario, Can.: Alger Press, 1984.
12. Jay, A. "The Meeting Chairperson: Master or Servant?" *Journal of Nursing Administration* (May 1981): 30–2.
13. *The A-B-C's of Parliamentary Procedure.* A Scriptographic Booklet. South Deerfield, Mass.: Channing L. Bete Co., Inc., 1980.
14. Jones, O.G. *Parliamentary Procedure at a Glance, New Enlarged and Revised Edition.* New York, N.Y.: Hawthorn/Dutton, 1971.
15. National Association of Parliamentarians. *Pointers on Parliamentary Procedure. Educational Material #1.* Kansas City, Mo.: National Association of Parliamentarians, 1984.
16. Diamond, E. "How To Conduct a Meeting." *Illinois Medical Journal* 157, no. 4 (1980): 236–8.
17. Patnode, D. *Robert's Rules of Order: A Simplified Updated Version of the Classic Manual of Parliamentary Procedure.* New York, N.Y.: Berkley Publishing Co., 1989.
18. *Robert's Rules of Order: Standard Guide to Parliamentary Procedure.* New York, N.Y.: Bantam, 1986.

Creating opportunities for employee participation in problem solving

Susan Kahn
Staff Assistant
Office of Human Relations
University of Massachusetts
Amherst, Massachusetts

O NE OF THE MOST prevalent messages in supervisory training today is that supervisors must be willing to allow their employees to participate in solving problems that affect them and must have the skills required to accomplish this task. Lack of participation has been shown to be a major factor contributing to organizational and personal stress that can have a dramatic impact on the health of the employee.[1] Employees who are given opportunities to participate in problem solving consistently exhibit higher morale and greater job satisfaction than employees who do not. Quality circles, one highly publicized mechanism for employee involvement, have received a great deal of attention in the literature on this subject. Studies have shown that quality circle participants, including supervisors, benefit in terms of heightened self-esteem, increased awareness of group processes,

Health Care Superv, 1988, 7(1), 39–49
© 1988 Aspen Publishers, Inc.

and improved leadership skills. Departments benefit because of higher morale, better quality, and the generation of cost-saving ideas. Also, another extremely important benefit is that participants in quality circles and other employee involvement groups learn an entirely new way of seeing problems—as something to be solved rather than simply complained about.

The article "The Importance of Japanese Management to Health Care Supervisors: Quality and American Circles," in HCS 5:3 (April 1987), outlines the benefits of quality circles and enumerates the difficulties involved in implementing them in health care organizations. After offering a convincing explanation about top management's reluctance to support such a complicated and expensive process on an organizationwide basis, the author states that "they [health care supervisors] must take the necessary steps to enhance employee participation within their areas of responsibility."[2] Unfortunately, it is at this point that most articles about employee participation end. Supervisors are left with serious doubts about initiating quality circles and with few, if any, specific suggestions about how to inspire employee participation within their work units. If there is not an administration mandate for organizationwide effort toward employee participation complete with intensive training and support, what can an individual supervisor do?

Is it possible for a supervisor to create meaningful employee involvement groups at the department level without being part of a top-down organizationwide effort? In an attempt to answer this question, consultation was offered to several supervisors who were then assisted in establishing several modified quality circles and employee prob-

These techniques can be easily learned and effectively used by supervisors and can have a dramatic impact on employees, supervisors, and entire departments.

lem-solving groups in a 450-bed medical center hospital. This article will discuss the efforts of three of these groups. These examples are practical guidelines for supervisors who want to implement employee involvement processes. The proven quality circle techniques employed by each of the groups, include brainstorming, decision making by consensus, data collecting, and cause-and-effect problem solving. These techniques can be easily learned and effectively used by supervisors and can have a dramatic impact on employees, supervisors, and entire departments.

CASE ONE: CENTRAL STERILE REPROCESSING

The first-line supervisor in central sterile reprocessing (CSR) was interested in starting a quality circle because of low morale and productivity problems in the department. The employees did not feel that they were particularly well regarded by the rest of the hospital. They complained about not being listened to and about decisions being made without their input. The supervisor hoped that through participation in a quality circle, individual members might improve their self-esteem and feel empowered and, thus, gain recognition from the rest of the hospital. It was also seen as an opportunity for "creativity amid boredom."[3]

The supervisor asked the human resource

department for consultation and sought the approval of the department head and administrator. The entire department (25 employees) was told about quality circles and, with encouragement from supervisors, 6 employees from 2 shifts volunteered for a term of at least three months. At the end of three months, if additional staff wanted to participate, two members would be added to the group and two current members would leave. Initially, the meetings were scheduled for one hour every other week. Members from the evening shift came in early and were paid overtime. Eventually the meetings were held every week because one hour every other week did not allow enough time for group members to come to feel that they were accomplishing anything. No time outside of the group meeting time was provided for training.

The consultant from human resources was the leader of the group for the first several sessions. She trained the supervisor and group members together in group process principles and problem-solving techniques while leading the group. (This differs from a traditional quality circle approach in which group members and leaders receive extensive training, often off-site, before the group starts work.) When no group member volunteered to be the leader after several sessions, the supervisor assumed this role. The supervisor was actively involved in the group but was not a member of their decision-making body. The supervisor helped to facilitate the process, made sure that one problem was solved at a time, acted as intermediary with upper management, reported quality circle activities at staff meetings, and made sure that minutes of meetings were taken and distributed to nonmembers and upper management.

During the first few meetings the group defined basic group norms. These included attending meetings regularly and on time, taking responsibility for self by using "I" statements, listening to and supporting others, and maintaining a positive attitude about the group. The importance of involving nonmembers in defining problems and in data collection was emphasized, as was the importance of distributing information about the meetings and giving feedback about input to nonmembers.

Through the team-building activity of choosing a name for the group, the consultant was able to model brainstorming, prioritizing, and decision making by consensus. The group then began work on identifying work-related problems. Through brainstorming the group devised a list that was amended by input from the nongroup members. The final list included the following problems:

- Space not being used efficiently
- Systems and processes used inefficiently
- Training inadequate or inconsistent
- Procedures not updated or complete
- Window area not consistently maintained
- Gas sterilizers not loaded properly
- Ineffective use of time when making trips to ambulatory services (in another building)

Two cause-and-effect (fishbone) diagrams were used to identify the major causes of two of the identified problems (see Figures 1 and 2). The group's recommendations about gas sterilizers were to

- rewrite procedures,
- train all staff in procedures and insist on consistent application,
- buy another aerator, and

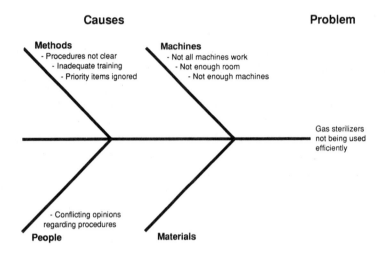

Figure 1. Problem identification: Use of gas sterilizers.

- use one sterilizer during the day and one during evenings, enabling evening shift instruments to be cleaned.

Group recommendations about trips to ambulatory services in a separate building were to

- establish central pickup area in other building,
- have exchange cart placed in other building, and

- ask personnel in other building to put items in a central location.

Through discussion of the proposed recommendations it became clear to group members that if the supervisor could arrange for the recommendations to be implemented, the van driver could pick up the instruments, thus freeing up CSR personnel. This realization came about only after a thorough analysis of the problem.

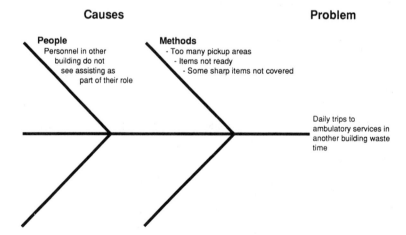

Figure 2. Problem identification: Daily trips to ambulatory services.

DISCUSSION

The quality circle in CSR met some of its initial expectations during its first year of existence. A number of difficult problems were solved, some procedures were improved, and the work space was redesigned. Recommendations made by group members have resulted in cost savings. Individual members state that the most significant benefit they received from their participation has been seeing improvements in their department. Members do not feel that their morale has improved through their participation. The supervisor feels that he has benefited in several ways. He has developed better group leadership skills through participation and is now aware of the importance of keeping the group on its task. He has learned a new method of problem solving and has found it useful, making his job less difficult.

The quality circle in CSR has had some problems. Nonmembers have not been supportive and have resented having to do extra work while members were at meetings, although nonmembers have been assured by supervisors that this is not necessary. Morale is still a problem within the department.

The circle recently redesigned the work space, and the entire department seems to be appreciative of this effort. One of the greatest sources of frustration for circle members was their perception that some of the solutions that they recommended were not acted on by management. (This is one of the most important causes of quality circle failures.)

Another frustration has been that no new members have volunteered. Several original members feel torn because they know that if they resign, the circle cannot continue; yet they are feeling "burned out" and would like others to take their places.

After a year the decision has been made to modify the quality circle into a problem-solving group. The circle will meet only when a problem is identified by either a circle member or by management and will stay together only until that particular problem is solved. Members seemed to be relieved by this decision because they were reluctant to give up the quality circle entirely, although they had run out of significant problems. This modified quality circle approach (a problem-solving group using the cause-and-effect method to solve already identified problems) may be a more effective way to create opportunities for employee participation in problem solving in the busy hospital environment than a traditional quality circle that demands a longer commitment. The next two examples will illustrate this technique of employee participation in problem solving.

CASE TWO: CARDIAC CATHETERIZATION LABORATORY

The department head from cardiology and the supervisor of the cardiac catheterization laboratory approached the human resource department for help in dealing with a morale problem that had reached a crisis point. A group resignation was imminent. A cross-training program, implemented several months earlier along with a four-day work week and the hiring of a new supervisor, was causing extreme anxiety and dissatisfaction. Much of it was targeted toward the new supervisor. The managers felt that they had tried everything to solve the problem and wondered if a quality circle might be appropriate.

The human resource consultant thought that implementing a quality circle at a time when there was such a big rift between staff and supervisor would not be appropriate. She agreed instead to an action research project with the staff, meeting with each person individually to try to get an objective assessment of the problem and then feeding back the results to staff along with her recommendations. It seemed critical to involve employees in any process that would lead to a recommendation for action. If the staff felt that their concerns were being taken seriously, perhaps a crisis could at least be postponed until a recommendation could be made.

Throughout the interview process, two problems were identified by everyone who was interviewed. (1) There was no schedule for nor consistency in the cross-training program, so some staff were inadequately trained and others did not feel comfortable working on a case with someone who did not have the appropriate training. (2) The new supervisor was perceived as not being available enough to the staff. He was perceived as aloof and not part of the team. Some staff felt that he was not supportive and that he did not value their skills. The supervisor and department head were responsive to this feedback, and the supervisor agreed to try to modify his behavior and to spend more time in the laboratory.

In the feedback meeting with the staff, the consultant shared the observation that almost everyone interviewed had a great deal of energy for defining problems but very little energy for generating creative solutions. When this behavior occurred in the feedback meeting, it was consistently pointed out to staff by the consultant. Most of the staff members recognized this when it

was pointed out. When it was made clear that management supported the supervisor and the cross-training program, staff members realized that it was imperative that they do some problem solving if they wanted to continue to work in the cardiac catheterization laboratory comfortably.

The recommendation to form an employee involvement group to address the problem as well as to provide a vehicle for team building was received more positively than had been expected. Because the staff had been part of the process leading up to the recommendation, most saw that the situation was hopeless unless they began to solve problems rather than just identify them. The recommendation for a problem-solving group was framed as an opportunity for positive problem solving and team building because the new supervisor had not yet formed a team with his staff. It was seen as an opportunity for him to develop leadership and group processing skills. An important part of the recommendation was that the human resource consultant lead the group, at least at the beginning, and remain as a consultant until a more positive way of approaching problems could be developed.

The group operated according to quality circle principles. Membership was voluntary. It was made clear to everyone that only those people who believed that the problems could be solved should volunteer. (All but two staff members volunteered.) The group met weekly and included the supervisor who took over the leadership role after a few sessions when the human resource consultant taught the cause-and-effect method of problem solving. This group differed from a traditional quality circle in that the problem the group was to work on had already been identified for them. The fact that this group started as the outcome of an action research project also made its process different from the process of forming a traditional quality circle.

The norms that this group agreed on were taken very seriously and included maintaining a positive attitude; discussing any negative feelings (particularly about the supervisor's behavior) in the group rather than outside; and prohibiting interruption by beepers or telephone calls. Negativism was not permitted. This was an entirely new experience for the group, and they rose to the challenge. It was clear that group members felt better solving problems than they did complaining about them. The role of the consultant, in addition to leading the first few meetings, was to monitor the group's process and to interrupt negative nonproblem-solving interactions. This provided a helpful opportunity for the supervisor to learn some different ways of interacting with staff.

This group analyzed the cross-training problem, using a cause-and-effect diagram (see Figure 3).

The group decided that the most significant causes of the problem were that no defined minimum standards existed and that the staff was relied on too much for teaching and assessing. The group sought input from nongroup members and drew up the following four solutions:

1. Define minimum standards and communicate them to everyone. These should be outlined by the supervisor and added to by the group.
2. Assess everyone on these minimum standards through the use of self-assessment and supervisory assessment. A form should be developed as the vehicle for assessments and should include space for follow-up.
3. A plan should be developed by the supervisor for remedial training.
4. A specific plan should be developed for the training of new employees.

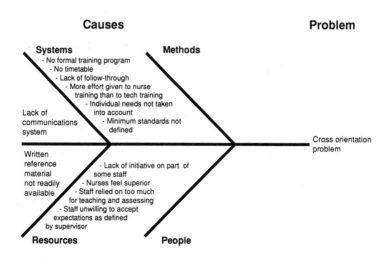

Figure 3. Analysis of problem with cross-training program.

DISCUSSION

The morale in the cardiac catheterization laboratory improved as soon as the employee problem-solving group was formed. The change in attitude of group members was remarkable. The opportunity to express themselves openly in a constructive way empowered all of them. The group functioned as a team-building mechanism. Members were able to see that the supervisor did have some good ideas and that he was open to their ideas. The consultant was able to point out the systematic pattern of the group—when anxiety in the department became high, staff members responded by attacking the supervisor who responded by becoming rigid and closed, which further angered the staff. The consultant was able to point out to the supervisor specific behaviors that triggered his staff's unfavorable reactions.

It was clear that group members felt better solving problems than they did complaining about them.

This group accomplished a significant amount of work in a short period of time. In three months a new assessment tool was developed, and each staff member had done a self-assessment and had been assessed by the supervisor. Staff members felt more confident about their skill level and the skill level of those they worked with. It looked like the cross-training idea, which was new to the hospital, would work. Physicians noticed the difference in attitude. Plans for remedial training were made, as was a plan for the orientation of new employees. Group members became committed to solving problems rather than just complaining about them. This carried over to staff meetings where group members were quick to chastise anyone not constructively solving a problem. Using the supervisor as a scapegoat virtually disappeared (except during times of high anxiety).

CASE THREE: RENAL DIALYSIS

The department head of renal dialysis was concerned because staff indicated on the yearly departmental evaluation that morale was a problematic issue. The department head wanted to explore this further and asked human resources for consultation on how to proceed. The consultant suggested that the department head use an employee involvement group to solve the problem rather than try to do this herself. This group would be given the responsibility of exploring the morale problem and recommending solutions. The department head saw this as a significant opportunity for employee involvement and agreed to proceed.

A request was made for volunteers representing the different disciplines in the department (technicians, nurses, aides). Six people volunteered. One supervisor was included as was a secretary. Meetings were scheduled weekly whenever possible. Some group members came in on their days off. The consultant from human resources led the group initially until one of the group members volunteered to be leader. Group norms were established, as were mechanisms for transmitting information to non-group members and to the department head. This group differed from a traditional quality circle in that the problem it was to work

Causes   **Problem**

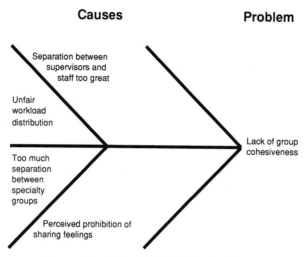

Figure 4. Analysis of lack of cohesiveness.

on (departmental morale) was already defined, and the group was time limited, that is, it would only meet until this particular problem was solved. It was similar to a quality circle in that membership was voluntary, the same techniques for problem solving and decision making were used, and data collection was an essential part of the process.

The group members met with nongroup members to discuss perceived causes of the morale problem. Discussion of this information led to the conclusion that the perceived morale problem was really a perceived lack of group cohesiveness. The morale committee analyzed the causes of lack of group cohesiveness as shown in Figure 4.

Each of the four main causes of the lack of group cohesiveness was addressed separately. The group identified solutions for each cause after receiving input from nongroup members. At the end of this process, recommended solutions were put on a form and distributed to all renal dialysis staff. Each person was given the opportunity to indicate the importance of each recom-

mended solution. From the results of this form, concrete actions were taken.

DISCUSSION

Participation on the morale committee was important for members in many ways. Besides developing group-processing skills and specific problem-solving skills, it was an opportunity for members to get to know each other better and to work together in a positive way, with a common goal, despite differences and conflicts that members had outside the group. Members felt good about the work they did, and this affected their self-confidence. They felt that they were contributing something significant to their department.

Lack of assertiveness had been a problem throughout the dialysis department. Group participation gave members the opportunity to learn to be more assertive because group norms included speaking up for oneself in the group if a member felt discounted, ignored, or interrupted. The group member who volunteered to be the leader developed confidence in leadership and presentation skills.

When the assigned work of the committee was over, that is, recommendations were made to the staff about solving the problem of group cohesiveness, the committee felt that its work was over. Members who had taken their task seriously and had worked hard felt somewhat burned out, and they wanted others to have what they considered to be a positive team-building experience. Another employee-solving group with different volunteers was then started to work on one of the specific recommendations— improving interpersonal communication in the department through training sessions. Again, instead of taking responsibility for solving the problem, the department head allowed employees to be involved.

Can quality circles work at the department level? From the experiences discussed in this article and from others not presented, it is clear that there are a variety of ways that employees in a hospital setting can be involved in problem solving at the department level. Modified quality circles, based on the principles of traditional quality circles but limited to one or two specific problems, can work well. This modification eliminates a cause of burnout described by quality circles members who have participated in a circle over a long period of time. It is also more manageable for a hospital setting than an open-ended type of group. Problem-solving groups that evolve out of an action research intervention, as described previously, seem to be quite effective because employees are involved in the process leading to the recommendation to form a group.

Supervisors play a critical role in identifying opportunities for employee involvement. By following basic guidelines and using the cause-and-effect method of problem solving, supervisors can involve their employees in problem solving in a meaningful way. Benefits from this involvement are manifold and include creative solutions to difficult problems, increased self-confidence of members and supervisors, improved team functioning, improved leadership and problem-solving skills, and improved morale of group members.

Basic principles that supervisors should remember when considering the formation of an employee involvement group include the following:

- Department head approval must be assured.
- Membership should be voluntary.
- Group norms must be established and should include maintaining a positive attitude and expressing any concerns inside the group.
- Problems should be worked on one at a time.
- Causes should be analyzed before solutions are generated. The cause-and-effect method of problem solving should be used.
- A consultant, ideally from inside the organization, should stay regularly involved.

•   •   •

Supervisors must be willing to be flexible about implementing employee involvement groups, and they should feel comfortable asking for consultation. Any employee involvement effort will succeed only if there is a commitment to act on and implement recommendations made by the group.

REFERENCES

1. Blanchard, M., and Taggert, M. *Working Well.* New York: McGraw-Hill, 1986.
2. Boissoneau, R. "The Importance of Japanese Management to Health Care Supervisors: Quality and American Circles." *Health Care Supervisor* 5, no. 3 (1987): 28–39.
3. Goldberg, A., and Pegels, C. *Quality Circles in Health Care Facilities.* Rockville, Md.: Aspen Publishers, 1984.

Index

Notes

Notes

Notes

Notes

Notes

Notes

Notes

Notes

Notes

Notes

Notes

Notes

Notes

Notes

Notes

Notes

Notes

Notes

Notes

Notes

Notes

Notes

Notes

Notes

Notes